Grant Writing Fundamentals Made Easy

Christine W. Hartmann

Grant Writing Fundamentals Made Easy

An Early Career Guide

Springer

Christine W. Hartmann
Department of Public Health
University of Massachusetts Lowell
Lowell, MA, USA

ISBN 978-3-032-35722-9 ISBN 978-3-032-35723-6 (eBook)
https://doi.org/10.1007/978-3-032-35723-6

This Springer imprint is published by the registered company Springer Nature Switzerland AG
The registered company address is: Gewerbestrasse 11, 6330 Cham, Switzerland

For my mentees

Acknowledgments Mentoring intelligent, tenacious, and inspiring individuals has been the greatest joy of my professional life. Many of them shared thoughts about and examples for this book. Their questions and early career realities sharpened its focus and influenced how I framed material. My gratitude extends to Marva Foster, Emily Franzosa, Michelle Hilgeman, Caroline Madrigal, Whitney Mills, Princess Nash, Victoria Ngo, Emma Quach, and Annie Yang, along with others.

My thinking was also strengthened by colleagues whose critiques, collaboration, and support informed my grant writing journey. Those who contributed directly and indirectly to this include, but are not limited to, Laurie Barrett, Dan Berlowitz, Barbara Bowers, Winnie Chang, Graeme Fincke, Sylvia Hysong, Vincent Mor, Christopher Sciamanna, Alex Sox-Harris, Kali Thomas, Renda Wiener, and Sheryl Zimmerman. Above all, this book would not exist without my research partnership with A. Lynn Snow.

At Springer Nature, the book benefited from the editorial leadership of Janet Kim, whose guidance helped shape its scope.

Competing Interests The author has no competing interests to declare that are relevant to the content of this manuscript.

Contents

About the Author

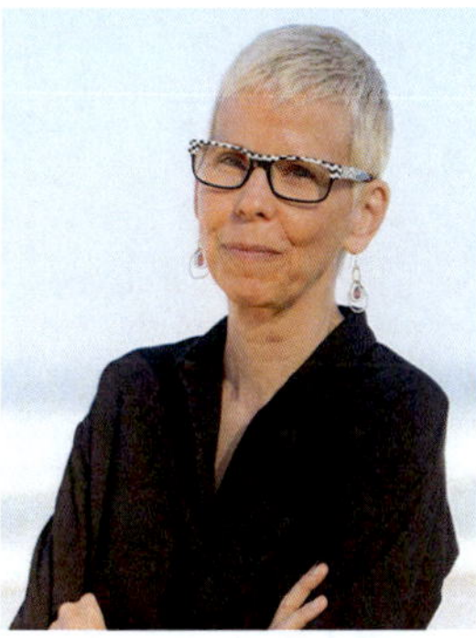

Christine W. Hartmann, PhD is Research Professor in Public Health at the University of Massachusetts Lowell in the US and a former senior researcher with the US Department of Veterans Affairs. Her career has centered on federally funded research, scientific grant review, grant writing, and mentoring early career faculty and investigators. Her scholarly expertise spans health services research, implementation science, quality improvement, organizational culture, long-term care, and aging services.

Dr. Hartmann has served as principal investigator on more than $20 million in competitive grants from the US National Institutes of Health and the Department of Veterans Affairs, including a Research Career Scientist award from the Department of Veterans Affairs Health Services Research Service. Her scholarship appears in numerous high-impact peer-reviewed journals. She has served on national and international scientific grant review panels, giving her direct insight into how reviewers evaluate grant applications, how proposals succeed or fail, and what early-career faculty and researchers need to understand about the review process. She has mentored early-career faculty, postdoctoral fellows, clinicians, and cross-disciplinary research teams, helping them secure more than $18 million in competitive grant funding.

In this book, she draws on decades of direct experience as a federally funded investigator, grant reviewer, mentor, and grant writing consultant to offer complementary perspectives on how successful grant proposals are developed and evaluated. Her approach focuses on helping applicants write grant proposals that are easier for reviewers to understand, trust, remember, and recommend for funding. In addition to her academic work, she consults on grant writing and engages in public-facing scholarship focused on improving research proposals. She is also the author of a memoir published by Vanderbilt University Press.

Chapter 1
Why You Need a Strategy

Imagine someone reviewing your proposal in the gate waiting area for a long-distance flight. This person had a day of back-to-back meetings, encountered rush hour traffic on the way to the airport, and stood an hour in the security line. They want a cup of coffee. Their eyes ache from squinting at the laptop balanced on their knees. But they have only 90 min left to finish your text before the boarding announcement. So they clamp on noise cancelling headphones and face your application with a grin-and-bear-it sigh, hoping for an easy read.

Did you give them one?

1.1 Cognitive Ease

My career depends on writing successful grants. Over the past two decades, I received funding as principal investigator of over $20 million. I helped write other proposals that brought in over $18 million. I participated in grant review panels across numerous national and international organizations. Each year, I assist with preparing many successful applications. I love everything about the proposal-writing process.

But I was not always a good grant writer.

As an undergraduate, I majored in German literature, with a concentration on the Romantic period, known for its convoluted grammar and heavy sentences that go on for pages. I embraced that style, mistaking obtuseness for sophistication. The denser my prose, the more educated I thought I sounded.

After graduate school, I joined a university department, where my department chair expected me to write grant proposals. Colleagues mentored me on how to develop a viable idea. But when putting it into words, my existing style clashed with page limits and expectations of clarity. Writing became a chore.

Then I authored a book on a subject unrelated to my academic life. The publisher assigned a professional editor, who redlined my text. I watched my sentences decrease

C. W. Hartmann, *Grant Writing Fundamentals Made Easy*,
https://doi.org/10.1007/978-3-032-35723-6_1

in length yet maintain their punch. I scoured the before and after versions of the manuscript to identify the techniques by which the editor achieved these miracles. But the methods remained a mystery.

So I studied books on grammar. I took classes to develop self-editing skills. Instead of thinking of my style as permanent, I made writing my hobby and tried to get better. Skillful writing, I came to believe, involved decent ideas, grammatical proficiency, and iterative revision. I endeavored to write proposals that I understood and liked. Yet few were funded. I wondered why.

I heard colleagues complain about the "arbitrary nature" of the grant review process. They felt they could not tell in advance what a committee would like. Reviewer scores were, at best, arbitrary and, at worst, rigged toward advanced or established investigators. Some exciting ideas received poor evaluations, and some lackluster ones secured funding. What a fickle process, they said, and complained about wanting to work in a more predictable environment.

Around this time, I picked up *Thinking, Fast and Slow* by Daniel Kahneman (2011). That book introduced me to the concept of cognitive ease and its opposite, cognitive strain. In writing, cognitive ease describes a reader's subconscious experience of feeling that reading is effortless, the written content familiar, and the arguments true. (See Chap. 7 for more about cognitive ease.)

Readers crave ease at the sentence level in the form of clear font, dark print, simple grammar, and well-primed words and ideas. They benefit from it at the paragraph and section level, with enough white space, logical organization of subject matter, and easily identifiable important points. Cognitive ease induces automatic, intuitive thinking. Reviewers who experience it are more likely to agree with what they see. Cognitive strain, on the other hand, unconsciously shifts a reviewer to a more analytic, vigilant approach. Readers who suffer cognitive strain are more likely to be wary, suspicious, and make errors.

Think of a proposal's text as a road. The writer determines whether the reviewer's drive is effortless or rough. Cognitive ease is like driving on a smooth highway with plenty of time and few other cars. It is easy. Minutes pass unnoticed. Your brain is relaxed. You enjoy the scenery and would recommend this road to anyone.

Then, suddenly, the highway turns into a construction zone. The pavement is uneven. Orange barrels signal abrupt lane changes. You step on the brakes. Your brain shifts to high alert. You expect trouble, hyper aware of further obstacles. That is what happens when logic, formatting, or other issues jar a reviewer, creating cognitive strain.

After learning about cognitive ease, each time I wrote a proposal, I thought about how the text would affect the reviewer, about what type of road I created for them. I looked beyond my content and edits and dove deeper into how to express concepts clearly. I leaned into what I knew about composition and strove to ensure every grant presented clear and logical arguments using wording that was accessible and easy to remember. I included key information early on about why the work mattered, what justified it, and how it aligned with reviewer and funding organization priorities. I focused on handing reviewers the material they would need during a review committee meeting to advocate for the application. Instead of writing for myself, I wrote for them.

This approach transformed everything. "For whom am I doing this?" became a driving question. The grant's objectives mattered. So did the background information, methods, team, and the project's potential influence on the world. But what also mattered—and perhaps mattered more—was how a reviewer might react to what I described and how I displayed the information they needed. I had to write for a busy stranger at an airport gate. That was the person who would judge whether my proposal was good enough to support.

That premise, I realized, formed the foundation for great grant writing. It was also the secret strategy to my consistent funding success.

Take a moment to picture your favorite streaming show. Most often, there is a team of writers behind it. And what is the one group the team does *not* write for? Themselves. Good authors never write for themselves. They might be proud of the final product. But the product was written for an audience that is *never* the writers.

Yet we forget that so easily. We author an email or a text message without any editing, understanding what *we* intend to say and forgetting that someone else might take a different meaning from our words. We also do this in manuscripts, crafting an introduction that states facts but does not hook a reader, because we, ourselves, are already hooked on our subject. We forget someone else might not be interested unless we explain why the work is important to *their* world. And we do this in grant writing, because the process is arduous and long. We spend a lot of time with the subject matter, with preliminary data, methodologies, and background literature. We eat and breathe the proposal's sections. In all that, we may forget the final audience.

How do you check in with yourself, ensuring you write a proposal for the reviewers? Below are five questions to ask.

1. *How do I determine if a piece of writing is good enough?* Do I ask myself whether the content is interesting, logical, or engaging and, if I think it is, do I tell myself I am done? Or do I additionally wonder whether a colleague would find the narrative compelling? Do I imagine strangers outside my field and ask myself if they would keep reading? In other words, do I write only for myself or practice analyzing my work from a distance?
2. *Do I test my writing on others?* Am I willing to share pieces with outsiders or Artificial Intelligence (AI) software? How do I react to others' opinions? Do I dismiss or accept them? (See Chap. 4, Sect. 4.5 for ways to have safe discussions with others about your work.)
3. *Do I avoid learning unfamiliar writing techniques because I have patterns that I repeat because I think they work?* Or am I constantly on the lookout for what engages me? Do I take note of how journal articles win me over with an argument or how an abstract creates a sense of emotional urgency? Do I try new styles in my own prose and evaluate how they resonate with my potential audience?
4. *Am I constantly looking for new sources of inspiration, maybe in unusual places?* Do I watch a thriller and wonder if I could incorporate a similar tension when writing my proposal's hook? (See Chap. 9 for more about hooks in grant writing.)

Do I analyze how a compelling news article drew me in, hoping to capitalize on that knowledge when I construct a grant's background section?

5. *Do I think of grant writing as a chore or an art form?* If grant writing is a chore, I will simply create reasonable products. I will not aim for excellence. And the final judge will always be only me. But if I view grant writing as art, I will grow skills to communicate better with my audience, hoping to construct a product in which they will recognize meaning. I will care about whether I am successful. I will continually hone my craft.

The script writers for your favorite streaming show create art for the screen. They work hard and probably enjoy their jobs. And their audiences judge them for their final result quickly and mercilessly, thumb up or down. As a grant writer, you create art in a different medium. You also work hard, with perseverance and creativity. Your product, too, will be judged. And if you embrace the process of proposal writing as artistic creation, you may also find joy in the journey, because when you craft text as a practicing artist you not only find new ways to share fascinating information but also tap into the best parts of yourself. And that can be its own reward.

As you analyze your position regarding grant writing, it may also be helpful to think about the avoidance-approach motivation framework from motivation psychology (Elliot, 2006). I think of avoidance goals in grant writing as those that try to prevent an undesirable possibility, such as, "I don't want the proposal to be rejected," "I don't want reviewers to find flaws," "I don't want to perform worse than others," or "I don't want to embarrass myself with an inferior submission." Writing a grant for these reasons may result in behavioral outcomes such as anxiety, vigilance, and cautious behavior. This orientation and these outcomes are not intrinsically bad. But they are worth noting if you experience them. In contrast, approach goals might be "I want to succeed," "I want to write the strongest proposal possible," "I want to impress reviewers," "I want to outperform others," or "I want my work to have a positive effect on the world." Writing a grant for these reasons might lead to enthusiasm, creativity, and persistence. Both orientations (avoidance and approach) can influence whether, when, and how you take the perspective of a tired but well-meaning reviewer during your proposal-writing process. Work to develop a sense of what motivates you and, if you realize you adopt more avoidance goals, consider trying an approach orientation.

1.2 Book Overview

This book is *not* about helping you identify or develop a research idea, scour the literature, or design a rigorous study. There are many guides that can assist you in doing those things. This book also does *not* exclusively focus on writing science, writing papers, or editing writing, though it touches upon each of these. This book is about convincing reviewers that your ideas are worthwhile, and that you are the right person to conduct your plans. It guides you in designing proposals that provide reviewers the information they need to argue on behalf of your work. The book's content applies to anyone developing grants. And it specifically supports early career faculty and researchers because they often find themselves struggling in the deep end of the grant writing pool. Consider this book a life preserver.

The information in the chapters is cumulative. I encourage you to read the book in order. That said, the chapters also stand on their own, with concepts repeatedly defined and referenced as needed.

Employ this book's techniques whether you apply for public (local, state, or federal government) or private (foundation, corporation, organization) grants. Use them if you are early in your career, preparing your first proposal, or want to improve your funding success rate. The methods pertain the entirety of the grant development process and across all types of projects and disciplines, from anthropology to astronomy, medicine to metallurgy, public health to physics, and seismology to social work. Navigating the funding world can be difficult and competitive. But by understanding cognitive ease, you have an edge.

Imagine two authors writing separate proposals with the same premise. The difference is that one author understands solely *what* and *how* to write. The other also understands *for whom* to write. Put another way, only one author writes for the audience.

Which grant writer do you want to be?

1.3 Use of Artificial Intelligence in Grant Writing

At the time this book was published, people still drove grant reviews and funding decisions. And people are, and always will be, influenced by how easy a proposal is to read and understand. If there comes a day when reviews and/or funding determinations are completely large-language-model-driven, those future algorithms will certainly also prefer a better written argument.

AI has value, even in environments rigorous about preventing the use of AI-generated content. At the suggestion of this publisher, for example, I ran the book's final draft through an AI copyediting software program. Of course, there is a substantive difference between copyediting and creating material. That said, many academic-oriented AI programs generate transparent and rigorous content. A key to using AI is recognizing what it does well, identifying where it falls short or produces inaccuracies, reviewing its products, and always being aware of any restrictions on its use placed by funding organizations.

The strength of AI is the recognition of patterns across vast volumes of data. But it does *not* understand what is intrinsically interesting or compelling. It only recognizes what it has been programmed to recognize. So its answers can be formulaic, driven by what it can access and the prompts it receives. Another shortcoming of AI for proposal writing is that it only incompletely grasps the larger context in which a work is positioned. This makes it a potentially problematic partner for generating grant text, which often requires a deep knowledge of legitimate source material coupled with a broad grasp of context (the field, unpublished literature and material from conferences or other sources, the proposal's environment, the team's past work, the review process, the achievements of review committee members, and the funding organization's priorities). Ideally, grant writing also incorporates a splash of creativity, which AI can only mimic.

If you consider employing AI in any capacity as you prepare a proposal, review the instructions first. Conduct an electronic search for the terms "AI" and "large language model." Understand what the rules are. AI for copyediting may be regarded differently than AI for text, image, or table generation. Using AI to draft a letter of support or review a draft of a proposal for logical flow may be fine, but using it to write a background section may not be. Identify whether the funding organization expects you to declare any use of AI. The more clarity you have around what is acceptable and what is not, the easier it becomes to employ AI to your best advantage, if it is allowed. If you are unsure, contact someone at the funding organization responsible for your area. It is better to ask ahead of time than to determine afterward that you broke a rule you did not know about.

The following chapters frequently mention AI. If you do use it, always check the work. AI tends to produce sycophantic answers, meaning that it will tell you what it believes you want to hear, even if that involves sharing incorrect information. Always ensure anything created or edited by AI reflects what *you* want to say. For an example of how AI can create problematic content, even when asked only to edit, see Chap. 14, Sect. 14.7. In the end, only *you* understand the intellectual context in which your proposal is drafted and how you want the words and presentation to influence reviewers.

1.4 A New Path to Success

This book represents the accumulation of over twenty years of proposal development and reviewing experience and over a decade of studying how to apply cognitive ease to grant writing. I have provided advice to academics and nonprofit organizations. I have assisted with applications to the US federal government, foundations, and corporations. I have led grant writing webinars, seminars, and study groups.

The approaches I share in this book describe a method I developed over time. Initially, I archived it in notes and through presentations. In 2019, I created a website as a repository for the strategy's main ideas, posting essays related to refining proposals. *Grant Writing Fundamentals Made Easy* represents the next generation of this undertaking. In this book's chapters, I share techniques for improving grant writing, along with real-world examples across disciplines.

Welcome to a new path to success.

References

Elliot, A. J. (2006). The Hierarchical Model of Approach-Avoidance Motivation. *Motiv Emot, 30*, 111–116. https://doi.org/10.1007/s11031-006-9028-7

Kahneman, D. (2011). *Thinking, Fast and Slow*. Farrar, Straus, and Giroux.

Chapter 2
Why You Need This Book

You write a proposal because the potential benefit outweighs the resource investment. But in anyone's life, intensive grant writing activities compete with other demands. Even small applications take time. Grants that award larger monetary sums often require producing long, intricate documents. And not all proposals are funded. The return on any investment always risks being zero.

You may have called on different experts to improve your probability of success. Perhaps you followed instructions outlined in other grant writing books. Many of these walk you through how to compile standard components of a proposal and give explicit guidance about what each section of an application entails. You may have attended a course that provided an overview of the entire grant development process. Manuals about technical writing skills might line your shelves.

Even after digesting all that, maybe you are still hesitant about applying or are nervous about a tough funding climate. Perhaps your funding success rate has plateaued or even gone off a cliff. You may lack role models and doubt your own abilities. Or you may want to apply for larger or more competitive awards. In any case, you worry your current skills are not up to the task, that other people's proposals will be more appealing than yours. You are unsure and cannot put your finger on how to fix things.

Any of this may lead to a feeling that succeeding in the grant writing world involves mostly luck and that the review process is random or even unfair. You may think you are in over your head and the effort to write a proposal may not be worth it. Have you felt worn out, scared, frustrated, or lacking direction? Such feelings are natural. I had them too when I began my career.

There is a secret antidote. What you have tried up to now may not have worked because existing books and courses rarely emphasize the importance of the *reviewer's experience* for getting a proposal funded. The deepest challenge of grant writing is not producing a fundable idea or fulfilling the standard expectations outlined in application instructions. It is knowing how to craft a grant that is easy to read and, therefore, convincing. A strong proposal smooths a reviewer's path.

C. W. Hartmann, *Grant Writing Fundamentals Made Easy*,
https://doi.org/10.1007/978-3-032-35723-6_2

2.1 Tough Funding Climates

Tough funding climates make the work of successful grant writing even more difficult. But you *can* still succeed if you understand what changes occur under those conditions and what to do in response. Here is what you need to know.

Resist Perfectionism
Striving to write a flawless application impedes success. In a tough funding environment, writing an outstanding proposal is important. But perfection is not. Every grant has its weak points. The goal is to discover and address as many of these as possible. We never find them all. Prioritize working on critical aspects and soliciting input from others. If you are a perfectionist or lean in that direction, find ways to combat that desire. Here are some starting points.

Limit how much time you spend on reworking sections you have finished. When revisiting a section you completed earlier, set a countdown timer and stop working when it goes off. Do not rationalize your way into spending more time after it has rung. If you must continue, reset the timer for a shorter period and obey it.

Enlist someone forceful and trustworthy to be your "no" person. When your draft is coming along nicely and you suddenly feel the urge to rewrite a large chunk of text, dive back into the literature, or revise your aims, consult with that person first. Tell them your ideas and, more importantly, what feeling is driving the eagerness to make the changes. Let them advise you and decide together whether the answer is "Yes, do it" or No, stop." Have them hold you accountable for the answer.

Set deadlines for sharing your work with others and adhere to them, even if you think your draft is not ready. Schedule dates for sharing in advance. When a date arrives, adhere to your plan. Trust that you had your own best interests at heart when you resolved to distribute your work. Be brave.

Be specific about what you need. When you distribute the text, indicate the draft is rough. Also specify the input you want. At this stage, do you need only big picture impressions? Or would you learn more from answers to specific questions? People appreciate having their energies directed in ways that are most beneficial to you. Believe that no one expects to read a "perfect" product.

Change #1: A tougher funding climate means more applications for every solicitation. This feels like a no-brainer statement. But an increase in application volume indicates interplay between two distinct factors. First, some funding organizations no longer fund or fund fewer grants, meaning individuals who would have approached them may look elsewhere. This pushes up the number of applicants at the organizations still in the business of financing projects. Second, this same shortage of funding sources also means smaller opportunities that were not on everyone's radar—or were not interesting to someone who was relatively confident about getting an alternative pot of money—may seem more attractive. This results in all funding organizations, large and small, receiving more proposals. For example, a niche professional society that last year had only ten applicants for a smaller career development award program might, this year, have 40.

What this means for your proposal: With fewer resources available, your submission will have more competition than before, meaning you will need to outperform a larger number of your peers. This is also a no-brainer statement, but read on.

Change #2: With more applications than expected, review committees may relegate a greater number to be streamlined (not discussed in full committee meetings). Not discussing some proposals is usual practice. Often, the bottom 20% or so may fall into this category. But if review committees do not have enough reviewers or time or if the overall quality of applications is deemed to be lower, committees may decide to spend time talking about only those proposals that have the greatest potential merit. In tough funding climates, review panels may decide to increase the percentage of streamlined applications, perhaps to 50% or more.

What this means for your proposal: Being discussed by a full review committee should be an application's minimum goal. For most funding organizations, this results in a score and a summary statement that describes the full committee's thoughts. If a proposal is *not* discussed by the full committee, applicants may receive only individual reviewer comments, or even nothing. And if you are not funded on your first submission and choose to reapply, less information makes reapplication more difficult. In other words, your chance of being funded on a resubmission increases when you can respond to what the entire committee thought were the main drivers of a non-fundable score. So this change in the funding environment also means you need to write a better proposal than before.

Change #3: Funding organization priorities drive more of the decision making. With additional constraints on the availability of funds, connection to funding organization priorities must be clearly identified early in a proposal. The review committee and those making the determinations about who receives awards must understand how the work proposed advances organizational goals.

What this means for your proposal: Proposals must link need, approach, evidence, and outcomes to what the organization currently cares about. This must be visible early, phrased specifically, and grounded in realistic facts. Reviewers and funders will see through grandiose claims. Provide them, instead, with details of how the project will result in credible change within the funding period.

Change #4: Reviewers have more to do. In a poor funding climate, everyone is busy, including reviewers. Due to the overall tension in the environment, fewer people may be willing to serve on review committees, meaning experienced grant review panel members may be asked to serve on additional ones or read extra proposals. For this same reason, other individuals who have little or no experience conducting grant reviews may be requested to step in. For them, the learning curve can be steep. Outside of reviews, advanced and mid-career folks may spend more time supporting early career faculty and investigators struggling to obtain their first grants. Or they may concentrate on submitting grants of their own. Or both. These commitments place extra burdens on their already full plates, resulting in less time to review applications. To the extent that colleagues leave or are forced out of institutions, more work falls on those who remain, causing a repeat of the problems already listed. All this means those who serve on review panels during times where money is tight may, despite their best intentions and efforts, have less attention and time to devote to their assigned reviews.

What this means for your proposal: Your grant proposal will likely be evaluated by people who have additional stress. So your goal—in this climate more than ever—is to make their reviewing job as easy as possible. You, too, may have more to do. But to convince tired but well-meaning reviewers, your proposal should be clearer and easier to appraise than in the past.

The critical part of any review is not only the impression of the individuals assigned to read the proposal but also the ability of those individuals to *advocate for the application* during the review committee meeting. Give reviewers maximum help for this. Answer review criteria questions early in an application, including how the work matters not only to the reviewers but also in light of the funding organization's current priorities. In the abstract, overview page, and other initial summaries, provide short, clear, understandable, and believable points that reviewers can employ during the committee meeting to justify the case for your proposal. Give them an argument to get behind and advance.

Change #5: Applicants throw more spaghetti (grant applications) at the wall (funders) to have more stick (receive more awards). Tough funding climates precipitate this "throw more, win more" behavior. In many institutions, faculty and researchers are expected to bring in grants regardless of rank or the prevailing availability of funds. So when faced with a shrinking pool of money, many decide that submitting more applications is the right course of action to continue, or save, their careers.

What this means for your proposal: Panic induces rash behavior. Advanced and mid-career folks may weather a financing shortage more easily. But those early in their careers are usually hit hard. Yet we can imagine what happens when, within a similar period, someone who intended to submit only one application instead submits two or three. The person gets less sleep. They feel more stress. And with more to write, they make mistakes, cut corners, and spend less time and energy on each application.

The "throw more, win more" idea is faulty logic. You cannot pick up applications and throw them. They do not exist independently of your time and effort. The quality of a proposal is *always* influenced by the resources a writer expends on it. Fewer resources result in lower quality. So when you submit more frequently or with less time than is optimal, you *decrease* your likelihood of getting any of the grants you apply for. This identifies the true state of affairs, namely, "throw more, win less."

The bottom line in a tough funding climate is not automatically to write more. It is to write better written and strategically prioritized and targeted applications. How?

Recognize when you are making decisions out of panic. It is difficult to stop panicking. But it is important to recognize when you do it and how it affects your decision-making. Take a breath and appraise your drive to throw spaghetti randomly. The condition of your application is an important component that helps determine its final outcome.

Establish whether other factors are driving your decisions. You may receive pressure to submit more grants from various quarters. It is not always possible to reduce these pressures. But they are important to understand and acknowledge as you assess what is best for you.

Document your own minimum expectations for getting a proposal into the "discussed by the full committee" group. What do you believe is necessary? What markers will you look for prior to submission to understand whether your proposal exceeds this bar? To do this, you will probably benefit from discussions with experienced colleagues. Write down any decisions so that you can refer to them later, because it is easy to talk yourself into submitting a less-than-good quality product if you lack criteria by which to judge it. Look at the tips earlier in this chapter for getting funded in tough climates. Generate criteria for yourself before you begin writing.

Realistically assess how much time and other resources you have and, given those constraints, how many high-quality proposals you can produce. Do this in whatever way feels intuitive to you. It may be a cost–benefit analysis or an Excel spreadsheet. Your goal is to determine what your life as it is now (not as you hope it could be) can support. Factor in issues from outside the work environment and possible resubmissions when you do this.

Prioritize proposals that will have the most positive effect on your career. These could be ones that give you more protected time, more money, a better position, or connect you with others who can help you. Scan the funding marketplace. Assess the likelihood of obtaining the grants that interest you alongside their application deadlines, requirements, and award size. Create an ordered list of your top choices, those that benefit you the most. Then decide which proposals to apply for and when.

It *is* possible to be funded in a tough funding climate. But to do it, you need to step away from panic and understand your own realities. Acknowledge that you, the reviewers, and the funding organizations are stressed. Invest your time and resources strategically.

Avoid the temptation to submit multiple poorer quality applications. Prioritize your energy where you need it most. Focus on what benefits you. Make the reviewer's job easier by using the techniques in this book. Proposals do not need to be brilliant. But reviewers require confidence that a proposed plan is worth doing and will work. If you give them that, you will outperform the panicked competition.

2.2 Story from a Tough Funding Climate

Years ago, an early career colleague wrote her first large grant in a competitive climate with a great deal riding on the outcome. Her draft proposal overflowed with text, far exceeding the page limits. She struggled with how to compress it. Everything seemed important. The editing task ahead felt impossible. Sharing the proposal for feedback required vulnerability. But the deadline loomed. I offered to help, and she accepted.

Because I had never read the proposal, I could, more easily than she, adopt the stance of a reviewer. As an outsider to both the subject matter and the text, I saw everything with fresh eyes. I stumbled over dense wording, was confused by unsupported assertions, and scratched my head at redundancies and logic gaps. My colleague, on the other hand, understood the proposal's larger goals, its methods, and how the proposed study advanced the science of her field.

So we worked together, reviewed material, and decided what to cut and where to add. We drafted, edited, and rewrote sentences, paragraphs, and sections to communicate the proposal's arguments without jargon and at the right level of scientific sophistication. We supported a reviewer's cognitive ease with a clear and logical flow from beginning to end. We added white space, graphics, and many headings. We aimed to have the final product convey a compelling, believable narrative that was easy to understand and defend.

We do not know under what conditions reviewers read the proposal. Maybe they slept well the night before, had few competing demands on their time, and had coffee on hand. Or maybe neighbors had a loud party until three in the morning, their boss emailed with an urgent request, and they left their coffee in the car. Perhaps they were at an airport. Whatever the case, we believe they found the proposal compelling and easy to read.

It was funded on its first submission.

Chapter 3
Tips for Early Career Applicants

Being an early career faculty member or researcher is demanding. Most mentors and advisors want to help. But often they forget to share at least some of the following information.

Money matters a lot. If you feel pressure to choose between writing a grant as principal investigator (leads to potential money) and authoring a first-authored paper (leads to potential prestige), write the grant. For outsiders interested in learning more about your career, a journal article occupies a line or two on your curriculum vitae; each grant in which you are involved occupies multiple lines: funding organization and grant number, title, role, dates of the award, and the amount. Articles, even those in top journals, require time to change the world. But your being principal investigator on a grant immediately assures others that intelligent people thought your ideas were worth financing. That builds cachet. It also provides you with an avenue to pursue interesting ideas and further funding, because project results can bolster the case for doing more work, and the more grants you write, the better at grant writing you can become, increasing your chances of success.

In the beginning, size does not matter. Early in a career, if you apply for the same awards that experienced colleagues or mentors pursue, you may not succeed. Yet having successfully competed for funding frequently matters more than the size of an award. Of course, a $50,000 grant looks better on a curriculum vitae than a $5,000 one. But reviewers and promotion committees may not care about an extra zero as much as they care about a history of success. Before applying, assess the likelihood of winning a grant. Also clarify for yourself the next step a grant can help you achieve: a dataset for a larger proposal, a collaboration, or a publication you can cite. Not every grant-funded project has to change the world, but each should produce something to reference in your next application. Even a small pot of money can function as a springboard, particularly if the project built on it produces tangible outcomes.

Learn how to write. Then, get better. We all learned about writing in our early school years. We may also have taken writing classes in college, graduate school,

C. W. Hartmann, *Grant Writing Fundamentals Made Easy*,
https://doi.org/10.1007/978-3-032-35723-6_3

or beyond. But how many of us study writing alongside our work as faculty or researchers? If we do not, we should.

Studying writing is easy. It can involve nothing more than rereading the first paragraph of a manuscript, news article, or social media post that captures your interest and paying attention to the content of the introductory sentences and the final ones. What techniques did the author use to engage you? Why did you find the piece memorable? What questions or emotions did it raise in you? If you practice analyzing writing that pulls you in, patterns will emerge. Then you can study what happens when you mimic these in your own writing. In short, approach writing as a hobby that requires continual improvement instead of as a skill that, once developed, you never need to revisit.

Competence and gratitude do not always mix. I continually meet terrific early career folks who would be farther along if they were not so grateful. Yes, early in a career, any offer of support or collaboration can feel like a leg up. Imagine you are in a postdoctoral fellowship, and a prominent colleague offers you an opportunity to serve as a co-investigator on a large proposal. The colleague says you have just the expertise they are looking for. If you have never been a co-investigator before, you may feel grateful and accept the offer. But if you are simultaneously working on your own papers and grants, this "opportunity" could entail considerable cost. You might spend more effort on their project than your own. You may not be involved in decisions about who does what or who receives credit for what, because their goals and motivations are different from yours. Even if you are promised authorship on manuscripts or use of data from the project to develop your own proposals, these things take time. In other words, a grateful "yes" can reduce the speed at which you accelerate your own career trajectory.

Every person who thinks you are competent and makes you an offer benefits from your saying yes. Think critically and carefully about what they gain and balance that with your own potential rewards. Competent people like you will receive numerous offers over the course of a career. Sometimes your immediate future profits more when you respond with something like, "I am grateful but must decline because of competing obligations. Please keep me in mind for future opportunities."

Everything has a secret code. Do not assume you know it. If you apply for funding from a particular source, nothing beats speaking with colleagues who have a successful track record with that organization. They can point out subtleties in the application process that you may miss or that are not explicated in instructions but are valued by reviewers. The same goes for all components of the application. Before assuming you understand what to do and how to do it, always look at examples and speak with those who have experience. (For more on Secret languages, see Chap. 7.)

Bad mentors may look good (to you). Poor mentors rarely look bad on the surface. They often have trappings of success: large numbers of publications and/or funded projects, a history of collaboration, and many staff and mentees. They may have won awards, including mentorship awards. But bad mentors can be dangerous. And it is worth knowing how to tell one from afar.

If you do not trust your judgment, and no one speaks up about whom to avoid, keep the following litmus test in mind. If you spend more time thinking or talking about how to manage a mentor's emotional reactions than you spend interacting with that person, you might want to distance yourself from them.

Other clues? Look hard at their curriculum vitae or resume, particularly the parts that indicate collaborations, such as grants or publications. Do they consistently collaborate with the same *advanced career* people, those who have choices about whom to work with? Or is it one grant or publication, and then that collaborator disappears from the curriculum vitae, to be replaced with someone else, who then also quickly disappears? Have they switched positions or academic affiliations more than usual? These signs represent warning signals—your job is to assess whether there is actual danger.

If you feel comfortable, ask their current colleagues or bosses, "Can you see yourself working with XYZ five years down the line?" If you speak with former colleagues or staff members who are no longer in positions beholden to the person, ask, "Looking back, is there anything you would have done differently?" Do not expect others, even those now removed from the person, to lay their experiences on the table for you to scrutinize. Avoid questions that back them into a corner. Instead, keep your eyes open for clues in body language, tone, and word choice. Recognize how these individuals would respond about someone with whom they enjoyed working. And absorb subtleties like lack of enthusiasm, a change in subject, or evasion. (See Chap. 6, Sect. 6.1 for more on mentors.)

Study successful colleagues' curricula vitae (by year). Documents summarizing careers accentuate both general trends and unique paths. Roads to success are interesting and varied. Identify what intrigues, motivates, or educates you. When you study curricula vitae, you also see how the relative value and function of papers and grants can change over time, how authorship on papers often evolves (from middle author to first author to last author), and how roles in grants are likely to shift (for example, from co-investigator to principal investigator or member of an expert panel). If you know anything about what happened in the lives of these individuals *outside* work, you may notice that career productivity often correlates inversely with events and stressors in people's personal lives. Moving, having a child, or a parent suddenly requiring caregiving can translate to fewer papers published, a downshift in work responsibilities, or fewer grants written. You may also notice that some individuals perform at the pinnacle in their field despite never completing postdoctoral fellowships. Some have a single focus for their research, while others excel in several areas. Some teach while others avoid it. Almost anything is possible. The key is to understand the main drivers of success as your world defines it and then to choose your path to success as *you* define it.

Performance matters more than prestige. When searching for a mentor or collaborator, keep in mind that what they do for you (actually do, not *say* they will do) outweighs how that person looks on paper. If you write a proposal with them, for example, do they participate in editing sections that pertain to their area of expertise? Meaningful participation such as this plays a much larger role in funding success than whether someone has an outstanding curriculum vitae. Involvement in crafting an application, not fame, improves quality. If a submitted proposal has glaring gaps that a person with an amazing reputation should have caught, reviewers will question not only that person's investment in the project but also how much they would be involved if it were funded. Lack of engagement can easily negate the weight accorded to reputation and stature.

If you want to boost your own productivity, collaborate with colleagues whom you trust to share some of the proposal-writing burden. Ensure their needs as well as yours are met by having open and honest discussions as early as possible about expectations. Continually revisit their involvement to ascertain whether and how you can improve the relationship. Chapter 3, Sect. 3.4 contains more information on collaborations and partnerships, which may help. Your goal is to foster a sense of mutually beneficial investment in pushing a proposal ahead.

Remember what I said about money? Early in your career, let the path to money drive most of your decisions. You have time for everything else later. Require data to generate more first-authored publications? Get funded to do work to give you something to write about. Want to buy your way out of a course? Bring in a grant to share money with your institution. Does your reputation need a boost or more publicity? Obtain a competitive grant award and publicize your success. Looking to support staff or purchase lab equipment…well, you have the idea.

Grant money cannot buy you love. But your career will certainly love what grant money can buy you.

3.1 Respond to Funding Organizations' Priorities

Before picking up a proposal, reviewers may never have thought about a certain subject. Yet after they begin reading, they should immediately understand why the subject is important to their world. That is the writer's task: hooking the reviewer by clearly identifying what and how will change if the application is funded. (See Chap. 9 for more on hooks.) This includes the effect on issues the funding organization cares about. Each organization has its own mission, priorities, and goals. It assembles review panels according, in part, to those concerns. A proposal's project and ideas must fit within all this; it must relate to the entirety of the context.

Always familiarize yourself with a funding organization's objectives. Because priorities shift, substantiate any assumptions older than a few months. Stay current. Analyze not just calls for applications but strategic plans, budget language, initiatives, and recently funded awards. Frame your ideas within the present context. Show the funder that the work will both advance the state of knowledge intellectually and the project's area in practice.

For example, imagine that an organization generally interested in patient-centered communication has a solicitation centered on improving communication among pediatric patients, their parents, and clinicians. An adequate application will indicate how its project relates to these subjects and will advance science. An *ideal* proposal will also position the proposed work within the solicitation *and* the organization's current priorities. In the case of the prior example, imagine the organization has a three-year campaign to "elevate children's voices." A strong proposal might build into its research plan the evaluation of different methods for soliciting children's opinions and indicate how this is timely and novel. When doing this, they might employ some of the same language the funding organization uses. Or an application might propose analyzing the effect of parental stress on children's responsiveness to communication efforts and how this will be measured to improve future studies involving children's opinions. The options for how to respond well are endless. A proposal writer's goal is to convince reviewers and funding organizations that, whatever the project, it addresses high-priority concerns.

To save time or in tough funding climates, some writers may attempt to reuse a proposal written for one organization in response to a solicitation from a different one. Yes, finding funding organizations with aligned priorities can help extend work across diverse pots of money. But because a well-crafted proposal has an argument and corresponding methods designed for a particular audience, this does not always work. It certainly rarely succeeds without diligence to ensure that the second application does not contain erroneous references to unrelated topics or to issues out of the scope of the second organization's interests.

Recycling ideas across funding sources requires finesse and great care to avoid backlash. When in doubt, give the summary or other early pages, *with all references to the name of the funding organization removed*, to a colleague (or AI). Have them guess the funding organization to which you are applying. They should get this right.

3.2 Filling a Gap is not Enough

Proposals must do more than simply fill a gap in the existing knowledge base. My bachelor's degree thesis dissected how three works of German literature from different centuries employed the motif of a mermaid falling in love with a mortal man and how the framing and content of the stories reflected each society's general stance on the position of women. Was this a gap in the knowledge base? Yes. Was it interesting to anyone but me? Probably not. It was fine under those circumstances. But the "interesting to me" approach does not serve a grant.

Human understanding is riddled with gaps. Has anyone evaluated the rate at which different breeds of dogs lose their eyelashes? Do we know the fastest speed at which a playground carousel can spin in outer space? We do not know many things in the world because we do not care about everything equally.

External and internal pressures can contribute to our thinking that a subject will excite others simply because it excites *us*. Undergraduate and even graduate degree programs may foster a sense that our own ideas have worth because we think them. Paradoxically, these predispositions can lead to our *underselling* the importance of a proposal's work or skipping over background information or details that would be essential for someone unfamiliar with the issues. It can also lead to assuming a reviewer (and funding organization) will be sympathetic because we think the idea is great, instead of assuming that interest is created through a clear narrative that is easy to understand and believe.

Advice about how to write grants often emphasizes showing the reader a gap that the proposal will fill. But effective proposal writing is grounded in principles that emphasize more than that. Yes, a hole needs to exist. A strong writer also crafts an application around the reviewer's world and shows the reviewer—with concrete and compelling facts that speak to the full context of the review—why they should care about supporting the proposal for *this* solicitation and *this* funding organization. Do not expect they will care. *Make* them care.

3.3 Assume You Are Overconfident

Confidence is a beautiful thing. You feel empowered, competent, and calm. But overconfidence makes you feel the same way. So unless you have experience, it is difficult to tell the difference. This underscores the importance of having your grant writing plan anticipate emergencies. Here are five questions to protect you from the disaster that can arise from overconfidence.

1. *Do you have experience submitting the kind of grant you are applying for?*

Yes? Then you understand all the moving parts and may have a reasonably accurate sense of how much time each part will take. To play it safe and ensure the grant you submit is the best it can be, your timeline may still need wiggle room for the unexpected: a brief illness, a colleague who does not respond when asked, or unanticipated competing demands. If you thought the submission would take six weeks of consistent attention, for example, you can build your schedule around seven or eight weeks, just in case. But because you have experience with all aspects, you do not require big buffers.

No? You will have difficulty predicting how long the proposal development process requires. You must collect information about all the parts, understand the guidelines, and assemble components that are new to you. In addition to the unexpected issues that can arise for anyone, anticipate the consequences of your own lack of knowledge. It is tempting to be overconfident and envision an ideal future. "I've done similar tasks before, so this will be easy." Or, "I am good at writing, so it will be quick." But if you lack experience, it is hard to tell when you are right and when you are (far) wrong. An overly optimistic stance can lead to last-minute scrambling and a poor-quality application.

When I submit for a new-to-me type of grant, I assume it will require double the amount of time than for a type I am familiar with. If I can usually finish a proposal in six weeks, I block twelve on my calendar.

2. *Do you have considerable experience writing and submitting grants?*

Yes? Then you can assess your needs based on past events. Look at your prior timelines and identify surprising obstacles you encountered. Can you predict anything unusual for the current submission? Allot your effort based on a worst-case scenario.

There is no danger in that. If you are done early, you can submit early. And relax early.

No? Assume you are overconfident about everything. Double, triple, or quadruple the time you predict an element will require. I know that sounds crazy. But here is an analogy. Where would the elevator business be if even a few elevators crashed to the ground? Nowhere good. That is why a *single* elevator cable is designed to hold all of a cab's maximum weight. And most new passenger elevator cabs are held by *four or more cables*. Why be so generous with extraneous cables? Because companies want to avoid any chance of a fall. Similarly, where will your proposal be if you hit the deadline before you are ready? Nowhere good. So arrange your submission agenda with extra "elevator cables" (time) to carry the weight of any prediction errors. Your process will be less stressful and more successful.

Start Early: Even YOU!

For those writing their first large proposal, every grant writing resource has the same advice: give yourself more time than you think you will need. But it is difficult to change your behavior based on what you read. You think, "I'm not like everyone else," "I have experience writing similar things. This won't be much different," or "I can't afford to spend that much effort on this. It will just have to fit into the time I have." You are not the first person to think this way, and you are not the last. But every early career person I know ran out of time writing their first large grant because they did not follow this advice.

The iterative process of proposal writing—where you share a draft, receive comments, rewrite, share again, learn more, and rewrite—caught them by surprise. They thought small administrative pieces would finish faster than they did. They did not anticipate that collaborators or letter writers would be less than optimally responsive. They got sick and had to take a week off. They hoped for help they did not receive. They thought internal submission deadlines were flexible. The list of things that can go wrong for anyone submitting a grant is long. The list of things that can happen when an early career person writes their first large grant is endless. The only way to control an unforeseeable situation is to allot yourself more time.

I repeat this advice throughout the book (see, for example, the introduction to Chap. 5). The repetition is intentional. I understand change is hard. I hope that the message will sink in by reading about various examples in assorted contexts relating to different steps of the application process. But you do not need to believe me. Ask around. Talk with experienced colleagues. Corral people at conferences. You will hear the same thing: my first large grant submission required much more time than I predicted it would.

3. *Do you know your collaborators well and have worked with them?*

Yes? Then you know who is dependable, deadline-adherent, and willing to lend a hand. And you have an idea of who overpromises, frequently turns materials in late, or avoids shouldering heavy lifts. You recognize that for those who are overbooked, you must get on their calendar early and develop an explicit plan with concrete dates for when to meet or give them drafts for review (and by when they will return them to you). For those who exceed stated timelines, you set artificially early due dates to ensure you have breathing space. And you do not rely on those who will not contribute.

No? You face a black box. Be careful. Some people do what they say, by the date you give them. Others do not. Hope your colleagues will be reasonably responsive. And include extra time in case they are not.

4. *Do you have experienced assistance you can count on?*

Yes? Terrific. Your proposal submission process will be easier because of it. Collaborate to set mutually agreeable deadlines. Then, try to share materials in advance. This is not only respectful but also helps if you run into unexpected issues.

No? Since you will have to shoulder much of the preparation and submission burden yourself, parse administrative and other tasks out for yourself, instead of saving them all until the end, when you may scramble and rush. (More on avoiding last-minute rushes in Chap. 3, Sect. 3.3). Create an overarching checklist that includes all components, large and small, to identify less time-intensive tasks to squeeze in when you have short free intervals. Working on smaller pieces in increments will also gradually result in understanding how much effort the bigger pieces require.

5. *Are you good at predicting how long things take you?*

Yes? Then use the overall submission checklist to create a timeline according to what you know you can do, increasing the allocation for each large task by a small amount, to prepare for the unexpected.

No? As indicated earlier, keep track of the effort you expend on smaller tasks to assess the commitment involved for larger ones. If writing a paragraph of your budget justification requires fifteen minutes (because you must check biographies and confirm budget numbers), then count all the paragraphs in your budget justification to estimate the time expenditure for creating the whole document. The same stands true for letters. Or sections for the proposal's background section. Learn from your past experiences, even if those experiences are all within one submission.

Stepping into a modern elevator is less stressful when you know that, if one cable breaks, there are at least three other strong cables in place. The proposal preparation process that accounts for potential overconfidence enables a more relaxed submission experience. It also ensures a better final product.

3.4 Collaboration and Partnership

Does your CV contain a section entitled, "partnerships"? Mine does not. Yet my career would not be what it is today without the authentic and meaningful relationships that emerged from collaborations and partnerships. If someone sifts through my publication and grant history, these are evident. But they are not called out by name, because a curriculum vitae has norms, one of which is to highlight the accomplishments of the author as though they worked alone.

But success is always the product of multiple brains. A bench scientist collaborates with people in their lab. A social scientist has co-investigators and colleagues. In industry, you create teams, squads, or pods. Some individuals collaborate mostly with peers, others with those whom they supervise or who supervise them. None of us works in a vacuum. Yet outside the realm of a formal mentor–mentee relationship, academia and science frequently shove collaborations and partnerships under the rug.

One result is that we receive little guidance on what form these relationships take, why they are important, or how to develop and foster them.

3.4.1 Collaboration

Collaboration centers on a unifying project or idea. In a collaboration, you join with a person or group to complete a task. This can be simple or complex, of short duration or long. But it is the project or idea that binds you together. How you collaborate usually depends on your role and the norms agreed upon by your group. If you are a co-investigator on a grant, for example, the specifics of your participation are usually ironed out at the proposal stage. If you collaborate on writing a manuscript, your team may have a publication and study data use policy (see Chap. 15, Sect. 15.3 for an example of such a policy), or you may hammer out authorship expectations as the idea takes shape. In any case, your role can differ from that of others, as team members often carry specific loads.

A fruitful collaboration may only last the life of one grant or manuscript. Paths diverge for many reasons. A collaboration can also extend across multiple projects or ideas, each new endeavor requiring a renegotiation of the arrangement.

Premature exit from a collaboration is possible. It need not derail the project or your career. It is usually not easy to leave in the middle because it may cause problems for other individuals involved. If you do it, be prepared that some collaborators may not respond well. If you must leave, explain your reasons clearly, without blaming anyone. I, for example, stepped away from a study on which I was a co-investigator because, a year into the study, I unexpectedly became principal investigator of additional studies. I cushioned the blow to the study and the team by finding a replacement for my position, which worked out well for everyone.

In collaborations, trust is helpful but is not a requirement. Sometimes you collaborate with individuals you do not know well or do not trust. If you do that, set clear boundaries, preferably in writing, and stick to them. This way, you can refer to agreed-upon arrangements if awkward or difficult circumstances arise. If you are in doubt about your fit with someone or a team, ask others about them or, if possible, begin the collaboration with a small project, one that does not involve a protracted obligation or much risk.

3.4.2 *Partnership*

Partnerships stretch over time. A partnership involves a long-term commitment. It is larger than a single project. It may involve the exploration of a scientific agenda that will encompass multiple studies and last for years or even decades. Or it may represent a commitment that is based on working style and other mutually beneficial aspects, independent of a single, shared agenda. Regardless, when you are in a partnership, you are in it for the long haul.

Partnerships in science and other disciplines, as in romance, are all about the individuals. Partners can be "two peas in a pod." Or the partnership can be a case of opposites attract. Partners may bring distinct, complementary strengths to the relationship. Or they may have differing perspectives or connections that are symbiotic. Outsiders need not understand what makes a partnership click. The partners know and appreciate that they perform better together than alone.

Partnerships are based on trust. Without trust, a partnership fizzles. Because of the long-term nature of the relationship and the commitment involved in striving for something neither individual can achieve by themselves, a good partnership involves a deeper level of trust than that expected in a collaboration. A shared understanding of what drives the value of a partnership is critical. This must be the product of honest conversations about priorities, pressures, and goals.

Partnerships are also mutually supportive. Because the commitment is strong, who does what or who pulls the heavier load can shift, according to need and desire. Partnerships may not hammer out all details in writing or for every project, because the partners understand each other well enough to be flexible and adjust expectations and responsibilities as situations change.

Partnerships elevate all parties' careers (and a contentious break up can derail them). A partnership may be more or less fruitful. But the goal is always that the relationship brings each partner benefits they would not have achieved otherwise.

3.4.3 *Why Are Collaborations and Partnerships Important?*

More brains are better. As noted already, none of us operates in a vacuum. The more people who contribute their genuine enthusiasm and intellect, the better a project is likely to be. And when you collaborate or partner, you can tap into others' networks. The wider their circles, the wider yours can become.

Not all collaborations or partnerships improve productivity, but most do. When you split the work and have support, your own tasks can become lighter. Avoid collaborations where the workload is unfairly balanced or you are expected to herd others into doing their jobs. These relationships are not fruitful, which is why it is always best to start with a small or time-limited project and gather information behind the scenes before committing to an unknown individual or group.

How can you develop and foster collaborations and partnerships? As I say elsewhere, try not to jump into a swimming pool with someone without getting a read on the water first. Discuss expectations up front and put them in writing. Consult with colleagues or AI and develop a plan for how to handle conflict professionally. Anticipate what to do if you receive pressure to take responsibility for a task you did not agree to, if you are pulled into a situation where you do not feel comfortable, or if circumstances or individuals impose themselves upon you.

If you join a group or a small collaboration, choose one with a leader you like. Ask yourself, "Would I go out for a drink after work with this person? Would the conversation flow easily?" If they are the director or principal investigator, do you like their leadership style? Do they treat their colleagues with respect? Do they have collaborators or partners whose work ethic you admire?

Not everyone moves a collaboration into a partnership. But building trust with a core group of collaborators can further your career. Keep an eye out for opportunities. And invest in relationships that matter. As in life, so in academia, research, and grant writing: it is not just who you know, but who you care about and who cares about you that can matter most.

3.5 How to Be a Good Co-Investigator

Being a co-investigator on a grant increases your research experience, builds connections, and potentially results in valuable pilot data or authorship on publications. It can also provide an opportunity to participate in proposal writing without carrying the entire burden yourself. Some colleagues may seek you out because they are familiar with your work. But are you also approached by strangers? Whether you are depends in part on whether you have a reputation as a good co-investigator.

What does being a good co-investigator during a grant writing process entail? Not as much as you might think.

Beat all deadlines. Deadlines represent the last possible day to get something done—this is *not* the date for which to shoot. When someone sets a deadline for edits on a proposal, send in your revisions as early as possible. This helps a principal investigator in multiple ways. They will not need to pester you. And if you "reply all" with your edits or put them in a shared document, it reminds other co-investigators to begin their tasks. Being early with your comments also gives the principal investigator time to respond to the issues and ask clarifying questions. This avoids stressful last-minute changes.

Letting the entire grant writing team see you as someone who responds early may gain you credit for future opportunities. Being on time is not always the norm. Many co-investigators do not meet deadlines. And people, when they have a choice, are likely to gravitate toward those on whom they can rely. So do not be the person who delays submission or causes unnecessary stress. Instead, be the one that makes life easier.

Contribute big picture ideas. Principal investigators are responsible for a lot of big picture thinking. It helps them when co-investigators assist. As a co-investigator, your distance from the day-to-day grant writing slog enables you to see things a principal investigator may not. Help refine the logical flow of the arguments. Watch for redundancies or inconsistencies. Add information to the aspects of the proposal in which you are expert. In other words, read the proposal like a reviewer will, with an eye to finding holes. And be gentle in your wording when you mention issues.

Offer solutions, not just criticisms. When you do find holes, suggest ways to patch them, even if this means digging through the literature or crafting new language. Show that you care enough to help craft a strong proposal. If the issue you find is too big to fix alone, offer to reread a revision.

Edit. If you are a good writer, offer to conduct an in-depth edit. In the world of grant review, as everywhere else, first impressions count. Not all principal investigators have a solid writing style. Even those who do can always benefit from another set of eyes. Tightening language is almost always welcome because word and page counts matter. AI can help. But, as noted in Chap. 1, Sect. 1.3, it does not understand the broad context. You might.

If you have any doubt about how your edits will be received, check with the principal investigator about what would help them most. Everyone's style is different. When you share your edits, be clear that the changes you made are only suggestions.

If the proposal requires too much work, I suggest editing only one paragraph or section. Problems with writing are often repetitious: convoluted sentence structure, careless typos, and paragraphs with poor internal flow. Highlight examples of what you find but only make edits on a few. Leave it to the principal investigator to review the entire application carefully or ask you for more help, if they want.

Help with small things. There are many parts to writing a proposal. And not every principal investigator has access to resources. If you have extra time yourself or think your staff might, check with those involved and, if they are agreeable, offer your resources for the principal investigator to use. Maybe you find formatting a proposal relaxing. Or you work with a person who enjoys helping with references. Perhaps you or others can write the first draft of the summary, contribute a list of potential heading titles, or proofread biosketches of other co-investigators. Be creative about contributions.

If you are an early career faculty member or researcher and the principal investigator is more experienced, consider whether they are someone you would like to work with again. If they are, be as helpful as you can without jeopardizing the trajectory of your own career.

Offer to help with other proposals. When the grant is finally submitted, thank the principal investigator and the entire team for their efforts. Tell them what you specifically enjoyed about the writing process. And, if it is true, include a statement about appreciating any future opportunities to work together again.

Being a *good* co-investigator requires slightly more exertion than being an average co-investigator. But your career may thank you for that additional push. And your proposal-writing teams certainly will.

3.6 Celebrate Wins

A grant submission, particularly one early in your career, may feel like you are a basketball player suddenly thrust into a kickboxing ring after only a week of practice. The experience is unexpected, chaotic, and painful. Afterward, you may feel exhausted, beaten up, or numb. You might also feel happy or proud because you did your best. And you almost certainly feel relieved to slip under the ropes and onto the arena floor, knowing it will never again be your first time. For subsequent contests, you will practice more. You will anticipate better, make wiser choices, and develop appropriate skills. You may eventually even enjoy the excitement of a match.

When you receive notification that your grant was funded, revel in the moment! Pop champagne. Go out for dinner. Jump fully clothed into a swimming pool. Do whatever makes you happy. But funding notification is not the only occasion to hold a party. Your career will also benefit from commemorating wins along the way.

News tends to dribble in: first your score, then the reviews, then the formal notification of award. It is not always clear when to hold a big shindig. Not to mention that notifications do not always bring good news. If you let a party ride on whether you receive a final "funded" or "not funded," your champagne may lose its fizz while you wait for the good news.

I suggest commemorating milestones within the overall process. I separate the post-submission timeline into four part: submission, score and reviewer comments, notification of a grant being awarded, and project kickoff.

3.6.1 Submission

Let your collaborators know you submitted. This includes mentors, co-investigators, other involved personnel, and staff. If you feel comfortable, share the final submission (many people choose to redact the budget and extraneous pages before sharing). If colleagues work nearby, invite them for lunch or drinks. If no one is around, host a virtual get-together. Grant writing is never a solitary endeavor. Do not make those who supported you wonder what happened with the final product. Acknowledge the help you received. Including your collaborators builds your network.

Mark a successful submission for yourself in whatever way feels right. Eat cake. Take a day off. Buy a new device accessory.

3.6.2 Score and Reviewer Comments

Most grant review processes involve one of two outcomes related to scoring: no score or a score. No score usually means your proposal was not discussed by a full review committee. In many instances, even with no final score, you will still receive written comments. This will provide information to use for a revision. This is a tiny victory. You may not want to celebrate not getting a score. But consider getting your team together when you receive the comments.

If you receive a score, try to avoid attributing too much to the number. Your score reflects a cross-sectional opinion of one review group. Certainly, a terrific score implies probable future funding. But a mediocre or poor score still has its merits. Early in my career, I received a terrible score on a grant submission and wrote an email to my co-investigators with the subject line: "They hated it!" The level-headed response in my in-box within minutes was, "You got a score. Not hatred." In that instance, my collaborators and I digested the reviewer comments when they arrived, decided to pivot to a new grant idea, and that new one was funded on its first submission. Think of any score as a steppingstone on a path to future success.

You may feel uncomfortable with the idea of celebrating a number, especially if it is not in the range you hoped for. But if you gather with your collaborators, the occasion can help build team cohesion and enable everyone to brainstorm next steps. Whether you pursue a resubmission or a new direction, you will often involve at least some of these people. Use the score and reviewer comments as an opportunity to regroup early and cement your team's sense of unity.

3.6.3 Notification of Successful Grant Funding

My research partner's former boss used to send a dozen roses to anyone who received a notification of a grant being awarded. Your boss does not do that? Send them to yourself. Or do what I do—buy yourself something you will use, something about which you can think, "This is my *successful grant thing*."

A funding notification is also the perfect moment to convene collaborators, whether you have gotten together with them before or not. Celebrate because you are happy the proposal succeeded. But also bring this group together to build camaraderie with individuals you will work with on a project in which you are all invested. A team functions better if they know each other. A party gives you the structure for facilitating communication.

3.6.4 Project Kickoff

Virtual or in person, the kickoff meeting for your grant should be an occasion. Think of it as yet another group party. For tips on what to do and why, read Chip and Dan Heath's book *The Power of Moments* (2017). Do not let the title lull you into thinking you already know everything they say in the book, because you are wrong. They present a compelling case for designing an unforgettable kickoff meeting.

Some ideas for how to do this include linking everyone to a larger purpose by making the project's subject matter personal and recognizing each team member for specific contributions that led to the proposal's success. You can also conduct a "pre-parade," a concept from another Chip and Dan Heath book, *Decisive: How to Make Better Choices in Life and Work* (2013). This type of discussion involves imagining potential positive effects of the project if everything unfolds in the best way possible. In kickoff meetings, I tend to use props to shift the atmosphere toward celebration, bringing balloons and bestowing lei. Whatever you choose to do, make the kickoff a defining moment for your team.

Research shows that humans remember peak experiences (see Chap. 7, Sect. 7.1 for more on this). We also tend to forget how long it took to arrive somewhere. Turn your post-submission milestones into peak experiences, regardless of the time it took to reach them. Develop into a principal investigator who excels at teambuilding. Become someone people remember and want to collaborate with. Construct a scaffold for successful project completion *before* you even begin the work.

References

Heath, C., & Heath, D. (2013). *Decisive: How to Make Better Choices in Life and Work*. Random House.

Heath, C., & Heath, D. (2017). *The Power of Moments: Why Certain Experiences Have Extraordinary Impact*. Simon and Schster.

Chapter 4
Before You Begin Writing

Grants undergo a review process usually involving individual reviewers who read and evaluate a proposal. Following this, there is frequently a subsequent meeting of all reviewers or, sometimes, people other than the reviewers. Depending on the funding organization, the number of reviewers and meetings varies, as does the meetings' order, attendees, and agendas. Similarities across the general processes, however, outweigh differences. Because of this, after every meeting in which I am a reviewer, I take notes on high-level lessons I learn about grant reviewing, which I share with colleagues, particularly those early in their careers. Over the years, additions to my list have grown fewer. That worries me. I wonder if, instead of understanding most of what I need to know, I am suffering from "the curse of knowledge."

As described in more detail in Chap. 7, Sect. 7.2, the curse of knowledge refers to the difficulty a person with a deep, intimate grasp of a subject has when explaining that subject to a novice. The expert forgets to describe key details, resulting in confusion for someone less familiar with the area. In the world of proposal writing, the curse of knowledge means that a subject matter expert risks alienating reviewers by leaving out necessary information. They do not see their own omissions because they fill them in subconsciously. In the case of my notes from grant reviews, I worry that I overlook issues that would help others because I am so familiar with them that they become invisible.

To test the theory of whether I fail to notice things during a grant review because I am overly used to the procedure, I spoke with a first-time reviewer after she joined a panel reviewing career development awards. Subsequent to the meeting, I showed her my notes and asked her to add her own insights. She immediately leaned forward with her first comment, "The review panel has a secret language!"

She was, of course, correct. No panel aspires to create a secret language. One of a review group's goals is to communicate its impressions to applicants clearly and succinctly. But each review group operates with its own explicit and implicit rules of behavior, has its jargon, and creates a unique atmosphere. My colleague pointed out

C. W. Hartmann, *Grant Writing Fundamentals Made Easy*,
https://doi.org/10.1007/978-3-032-35723-6_4

that our group frequently used the term "lack of mentor engagement" when summarizing impressions. For the committee, this phrase signaled that mentors should have been more involved in guiding the early career applicant's science because the application, as written, was not at the level of sophistication we expected for a mentored award. But my colleague felt the language was cryptic. She thought the statement could be interpreted in multiple additional ways. She pointed out that someone could read it to simply mean, "the applicant should write more papers with the mentor" or "the proposal needs to describe a greater number of mentor-mentee meetings." Her perspective was eye-opening. The panel members failed to notice the secret language because they spoke it already.

Whether you are an experienced grant writer or a novice, awareness helps combat the curse of knowledge, which helps cultivate reviewers' cognitive ease. The three strategies described here help you gain a deeper understanding of the system in which a proposal's review takes place. Revisit these each time you apply for a different grant because each funding organization and review panel is different, and what you learn for one type of application may not entirely translate to another.

4.1 Become a Reviewer

Serving as a member of a review group helps you write a better proposal. You learn about the process and responsibilities of reviewers, see different writing styles, and are exposed to other members' thoughts and attitudes. You learn the importance of having critical information front and center in an application. If you can serve on a panel within the organization you are interested in applying to, marvelous. But wherever you join, you will gain first-hand exposure to what reviewer cognitive ease and cognitive strain feel like and what causes each.

If you are offered an opportunity to participate in a review, consider accepting, even if you have competing commitments or think you do not have expertise or the right qualifications. If someone asked you, they believe you possess the necessary skills. As with anything, you can improve over time.

If you have never been asked to participate in a review, seek out possibilities. If the funding organization you are interested in does not have an opportunity, find something similar. Governments and other large entities often share information about how to join a review panel. Search online for the names of funding organizations combined with terms such as "grant reviewer recruitment" or "peer reviewer opportunity." Some programs have special slots for those who are still early in their careers. Fill out one application or a few. If you get multiple offers, you can decline some, indicating you would like to be considered later. Even a review process internal to your own organization can be instructive.

Serving as a reviewer means participating in a time-consuming process. Your schedule may already be packed. You might juggle multiple responsibilities. But convincing a reviewer in a grant application requires understanding what barriers they face. By becoming a hungry, stressed reviewer sitting at an airport gate with a neck ache yourself, you can learn how to keep such a person engaged and what that person needs.

To do so, take on two roles as you review proposals. One is that of reviewer: commit seriously to the process, bring an open mind to each application, and judge each using equitable and objective criteria. The other role is that of observer of your own experience: keep a close eye on any reactions, however slight, that are caused by what you read and find. This requires self-awareness. Not every reviewer immediately brings this to their work. But it is a skill you can cultivate. What moves you emotionally or tickles your logical side? How much does jargon, abbreviation use, and sentence length influence your mood? Observe how you react to dense text and no white space. How quickly do you discover answers to the questions the review criteria pose? Can you grasp whether the proposal aligns with funding organization priorities? What thoughts do you have about the proposal that arise from the ease or difficulty of doing these things?

Participation in a review panel represents your window into a special world. And once you understand how much a proposal's form and content contribute to a reviewer's experience, you can use that knowledge to improve what you submit.

4.2 Get and Analyze Successful Examples

Avoid thinking you understand everything about how to write a proposal only by skimming the published request for applications or other instructions. You would not try to assemble a bicycle from parts without a functioning version in front of you. Do not attempt the equivalent with a grant.

Many experienced grant writers never sit down to write without at least one successful example in front of them, no matter how sure of themselves they are or how little time they have. This is a good rule of thumb. You may not find one funded under the exact same request for applications. But you can almost always find one from a similar field or funding organization.

If you want to write an application for a large funding organization, there are often successful examples online. Search the name of the funding organization and "example grant application." The US National Institutes of Health, for example, posts entire application packages, courtesy of generous principal investigators who have shared them for public consumption. If you are applying for a mentored career development award, find one of those. If your target is a foundation, look through the recent awardees and see if you know someone (or know someone who might know someone) to ask. If you enlist AI to help you, ensure that you understand the sources AI pulled its examples from. Double-check whether they were successfully *funded* proposals, not simply submitted ones.

If you aim to apply for a federal grant in the US, the Freedom of Information Act is on your side. All federal proposals should be made available to the public in response to a formal request. But, of course, you cannot cold-email the leading expert in your field and say, "Under the Freedom of Information Act, I could get a copy of your recently funded proposal. So you might as well hand it over now." That is not the way to make friends.

Instead, appeal to colleagues kindly. You can also request that these colleagues, in turn, ask their friends, mentees, and mentors about their willingness to share. Not everyone feels comfortable distributing their own work. But keep trying. Someone will be willing. The proposals you receive may not perfectly fit with yours. But they were funded. As such, they are valuable.

In tough funding environments and those with a rapidly shifting landscape, the more recent an example proposal, the more valuable it is. You can use older applications to analyze style. But only newer ones will provide information on what an organization is currently interested in funding. Your topic will never be precisely the same as that of the grants you find. In fact, unearthing a successful proposal with a similar topic is often only useful to examine how someone applied a specific method or managed a common concern. Prioritize recency instead of trying to match your area exactly.

Once you have a few successful examples, analyze how the writers organized and presented their information. Read a proposal while observing its effect on you. What parts convinced you? What left you feeling bored or confused? Asking yourself these questions will pinpoint writing you may want to imitate or avoid.

In any successful example, also focus on how the writers achieved cognitive ease for the reviewer. First, recognize patterns. Not all funded grants are astounding works of art. Many have spots that shine. Some have entire sections or pages that sparkle. But most also have rough points. Read enough to recognize a moment of excellence when you see it. Then, look across proposals and find several where similar parts are compelling. Copy these into a single document or open them simultaneously and analyze how each author achieved this effect. Stay alert for tone and any sense of mounting tension to build an argument. Do the authors have a similar flow to their paragraphs? Is their organization comparable? Do they display data in certain formats? How do they ensure reviewers rapidly find what they need? This process may feel like going back to school. But getting better at proposal writing requires repetition, attention to detail, and interacting with people who are better at it than you. Strong examples are great teachers.

Next, recognize techniques. Once you discover the patterns that engage you, dissect them further to discover the methods by which the authors created them. This could involve counting how many sentences comprise a paragraph or the number of paragraphs in a section. What about length—do they keep sentences or sections short or long? Where is the punchline? Does every sentence have an assertion supported by data? What verbs do they employ? Is there any unusual formatting? Where do they put supporting figures or tables and how are data displayed? Can you identify what hooks you, where the hook is positioned, and how it is constructed? (See Chap. 9 for more on hooks.)

If you have great grants picked out already, this analysis can be quick. Focus on the same paragraph (the first paragraph of the executive summary or overview, for example). Assess them with a critical eye. Be open to anything that stirs within you. And write down particularly effective patterns and techniques.

Finally, recognize the stories. *Great* grants read like solid works of nonfiction. The reviewer forgets they are reading as the text pulls them smoothly from argument to argument. Time passes quickly. They experience only cognitive ease. *Outstanding* grants achieve even more. They tell stories. Their points are personalized. Data about chemical reactions, analyses, or methodological advancement relate directly to things reviewers and funding organizations care about. They use analogies to explain arguments. The narrative is a cohesive, closed loop, always relating back to the main point, always guiding the reviewer, without digression, farther along the path. Days after you read an outstanding grant, you can still summarize the primary argument in a few sentences. It sticks with you. Because it moved you, you know why the work is important after the details have faded.

Many grant writing books explain basic details of proposal development, foundational practicalities that are important to learn. But there is more to getting funded than having a promising idea and pulling the correct pieces together. The more competitive the environment, the tougher the funding climate, the more you need to find examples you love and read them as if you are reading a favorite book. Let their style, techniques, and stories sink into you until they become your own.

4.3 Understand the Review Criteria

Why do self-help books have chapters and an index and, for digital books, a search function? Because these make the reader's life easier. That helps sell books. Yet many people organize proposal content in a way that makes a reviewer's task more difficult. That does not help sell a proposal.

Prior to a review, a funding organization gives reviewers instructions on what to evaluate. These instructions are typically easy for applicants to find because most requests for applications list the criteria on which a proposal will be judged. The instructions announce something along the following lines: "proposals are rated on...," "scoring will use the following as a basis...," or "reviewers are instructed to judge..." If you can find nothing, email the contact person. Review criteria are not secret.

A well-written proposal makes it easy for a reviewer to find answers. If "innovation" is a criterion, include a clearly labeled innovation section. If "potential for wider dissemination" ranks high on the list, a reviewer should have no trouble finding out about the project's potential. Yet many proposals cause cognitive strain by burying such key information.

Some writers feel constrained because the instructions that come with an application outline sections a proposal should include. These writers are not clear on how to position all they want to say within an imposed structure. But instructions are usually descriptive, not prescriptive, meaning you should include what is required but are allowed to introduce other sections or create meaningful subsections. Sometimes, an application must be submitted via an online form, where the sections are unchangeable. Yet even within those more templated formats, you can create headings and otherwise mark answers to key points. Reviewers appreciate any effort to highlight what they need to evaluate.

Find a logical way to answer review criteria as early as possible in the text, including in an abstract or other early summary. If the section lacks space to add a heading, start a paragraph with a bolded phrase taken from the review criteria and follow it with how you address that criterion. If the criteria indicate you will be reviewed on the "experience of the team," for example, you might consider beginning with, "The collective experience of this team ensures the project's success. This team has...".

Make the reviewer's job simple. Avoid having them search for essential information. Instead, display it on a platter for them to use when they advocate for your proposal in a committee meeting.

4.4 Cultivate Critics

Prior to submission of a proposal, the person most likely to imitate a reviewer's reaction is a critic of your work. Learn from this outsider's perspective. Your mentors and friendly colleagues have your best interests at heart. But their supportive feelings toward you and your application may influence them to ignore the biggest holes in your argument. The principle of cognitive ease requires maximizing the ease for everyone, including someone who initially has a negative reaction to your project.

Know and respect your personal tolerance for critical feedback and understand that your tolerance can fluctuate depending on internal and external circumstances. Sidestep colleagues who unvaryingly make you feel worse about yourself and your abilities. Avoid sharing with individuals who cut you down. But once you have identified critics to avoid, keep an eye out for others who can help.

They are the colleagues with whom you may not interact much, who you feel are too exacting, or whom you have watched deconstruct other people's arguments. They may be surprised by a request from you. But when you need an outside pair of eyes, think of them. Section 4.5 outlines a technique for discussing your work that operationalizes a critical point: there is no perfect writing. Every grant can always get better or be written differently. Flawless sentences, sections, or pages do not exist. Your goal (everyone's goal) for a proposal is simply to write it better than the last time.

Getting input from others can help you do this. These are some of the individuals with whom you may wish to engage in a dialogue.

Advanced Career Critic This is someone who has much more experience than you, in general or in a particular realm. Usually, they pay little attention to you. Or they might applaud some of your ideas and not others. They may seem too busy to help. But people enjoy being asked for their expert perspective. An infrequent request can succeed. The worst thing this person will say is that they are too busy.

Envious Colleague Critic This person may be at your career level or not. But wherever they sit, they think your life is a little easier than theirs. The truth of that does not matter. What matters is that a colleague who feels disgruntled by your achievement is paying attention to you. This individual may jump at the chance to share their opinions.

Know-It-All Critic You know who these people are. They have a reaction to every idea. Even if you think they talk too much, keep an open mind. Do they say things you agree with? Are they prescient? When rubber meets road, do you value their insight? Do they have experience you lack? They might be just the person you are looking for.

Critic Who Does Not "Get" Your Work In their book about behavior change, *Switch: How to Change Things When Change is Hard* (2010), Chip and Dan Heath underscore that what appears to be resistance from someone may simply be lack of clarity. Sometimes a critic does not understand your work because you do not express yourself well. Your reviewers might feel the same way. Let the critic explain what they do not understand so you can edit to maximize cognitive ease.

AI Critic If it is allowed (see Chap. 1, Sect. 1.3) and you feel comfortable sharing your original ideas, engaging AI in a review of a section or the entire draft can be helpful. The more specific you are when soliciting feedback, the more useful this experience is. Prompt the software to act as a reviewer for the funding organization you are applying to. Ask it to look for logic gaps, what a reviewer might see that you overlooked, sections that seem unbalanced, or weaknesses in the justification, team, or methodology. Ask it to assess how and where you placed critical information. Does it know without being told what funding organization or solicitation this text responds to? Be precise with your prompts and do not accept its first answer. Require justification for its opinions. AI can help, but only if you engage with it as an imperfect tool, not a sage.

Substitute Critic If you cannot or do not want to use any of the other critics, ask one of your friendly colleagues to adopt a skeptical stance. Beseech them to take the perspective of someone who wants to critique your proposal. Your friends may need persuading to read your work through a rigorous, unforgiving lens. But you will profit from the extent to which they do.

A colleague who is out for blood is a person to avoid. But value a colleague who does not put you on a pedestal. Keep a list of people who have said things you did not want to hear, things that you later realized were relevant. Those are the critics who can help maximize your proposal's chance for success, even if they do not realize they are helping.

4.5 How to Have Productive Dialogues with Critics

Writing a proposal requires putting your thinking on display. At any point in a career, this exposure can feel daunting. But early in a career, when a great deal rests on the outcome, the stakes may feel higher.

This is even more reason to ask others to review your proposal before submission. But receiving the criticism implied by the term "critic" can feel overwhelming. How to gather feedback in a way that feels safe and productive?

4.5.1 Dialogues with Colleagues

You may want to delay sharing a draft with colleagues because you want it in a "better" state. But early feedback is often the most helpful. It enables back and forth about ideas and allows time for changes. Set a date and time on your calendar by which you will share your proposal, regardless of the state it is in. Then, do it.

The resulting conversations about your draft, whether face-to-face or written, are easier when conducted with the understanding that perfection is not achievable and no one has "the right" answers. To facilitate these discussions, I offer an adaptation of the four-step Critical Response Process described by Liz Lerman and John Borstel in *Liz Lerman's Critical Response Process: A Method for Getting Useful Feedback on Anything You Make, from Dance to Dessert* (2003). The book contains many useful details to help both you and a reader prepare for a mutually respectful and beneficial dialogue. I summarize Lerman and Borstel's four steps as follows: the reader gives the writer positive feedback; the writer asks the reader questions; the reader asks the writer neutral questions; and the reader asks the writer for permission to offer opinions.

The process works best if both you and the reader acknowledge the many ways people can react to a text. It also helps if you both appreciate each other's time investment. State up front that this process runs differently from how academics usually submit and receive feedback and may feel initially uncomfortable, especially to those who are used to expressing their opinions bluntly or perceive a moral obligation to share their "wisdom." Set the stage for the upcoming dialogue by introducing the concept of "no perfect application" *alongside* your commitment to producing an excellent proposal. You can help a reader prepare by sharing details of the process beforehand.

Step 1: The reader tells the writer (you) what they liked, positive aspects that stood out to them, and/or what they found convincing, compelling, novel, rigorous, or exciting.

Step 2: You ask the reader questions. These can relate to what the reader said in Step 1 or may be different. In this step, the reader commits to staying on the topic of your question. If you did not ask about it, they should not bring it up.

Note that this latter principle stands in direct contrast to the typical process of peer-review, where a reviewer mentions comments in their role as "expert." In the Critical Response Process, you, the author of the work, guide the discussion based on what will help you the most. It is the reader's responsibility to acknowledge that only *you* know what you need and to respond accordingly.

Both here and in Step 4, the reader may, consciously or unconsciously, turn the discussion toward concrete solutions to a perceived problem. This is usually well-intentioned. But it may feel uncomfortable to you, particularly because solutions are only necessary if there is an issue, and it may only be the reader who thinks of something as a problem, not you.

Before beginning, imagine a discussion that involves the reader offering you a "fix" to a "problem." Does it feel reassuring? Or does it feel like someone is stepping on your toes? Does having someone offer a solution before you notice an issue hamper your ability to recognize issues yourself? Or does it open your eyes to new ways of seeing? Find your own answers to these questions and structure the process accordingly.

Also think about how Step 2 (and the later Step 4) can help you investigate components of the proposal *without* the reader jumping to solutions. Consider using prompts such as, "Please confine your answers to my questions. I understand you may see other things in the proposal than what I ask about. But please respect my process for improving the application in my own way." If the reader raises an issue or poses a solution anyway, ask them to think about the opinion that underlies the issue or solution and have them (or you) pose neutral questions (see Step 3) around that broader subject instead.

Steps 3 and 4 are optional. Undertake them only to the extent you feel comfortable.

Step 3: The reader asks you neutral questions. Neutral questions are those that do not state or imply an opinion, a "correct" response, or a value judgment. They do not put the reader center stage. Nor do they put you on the spot. These questions may be, but do not need to be, about a topic on which you both can later collaborate to improve the application.

Examples of neutral questions are, "When do you wish to submit?" "How did you choose the methods?" "What message do you hope the reviewer will remember when they read the first paragraphs?" "What excites you most about the work you propose?" The questions can, of course, be more specific and targeted than these examples. But they cannot be leading ("Don't you think a change to your methods would benefit the analysis?"), imply the reader knows better than you or caught an error ("Why would you select the ABC method, since it's so overused?" or "Have you shown the analysis section to a statistician?"), or feel like a trap ("How can you possibly substantiate the XYZ statement in the introduction?").

Step 4: The reader asks for permission to state their opinions. It helps if the reader is specific about which component they wish to address when they do this, by saying things such as, "Would you like to hear my opinion about ABC in the methods section?" or "I have a lot of experience in the area of XYZ. I would like to offer an opinion that might help. Would that be comfortable for you?" You are free to say no to any of these requests.

The goal of this dialogue is to bring you (the writer) to the forefront of the discussion as leader of the proposal, to value your needs and vision, and to respect your judgment and boundaries. Not every person will be willing to engage in such a process with you. But a commitment to crafting a proposal in dialogue with others resonates with many people.

4.5.2 Mock Review Sessions

A mock review panel or mock study section, where colleagues function as grant reviewers in a structure similar to reviews conducted at large funding organizations, can provide you with valuable information. It can also feel terrifying, because even though it is the proposal under the microscope, you may still feel like the specimen.

But, as noted before, any comments you receive *prior* to submission may help strengthen the application, particularly if they are constructive. So the question is not *whether* to seek out a mock review but *how* to organize one that serves your own best interests.

The four steps described earlier that are adapted from the Critical Response Process can inform the structure of a mock review process. You might also do the following.

1. *Choose reviewers for the mock panel carefully.* Ask people who will take your requests about the process seriously. Select them not only for expertise but also for personality and collegiality.
2. *Assign tasks.* Have someone in authority (experienced colleague, department chair) serve as the timekeeper, to ensure that the mock reviewers adhere to the stated time limits for their reviews. In real grant review sessions, people going over their allotted time can be a problem. So make sure the timekeeper will enforce the agreed-upon rules.
3. *Consider having a facilitator.* If you do not want to facilitate the process yourself, assign one. Again, choosing a person with experience will help. Also assign a note taker, or transcribe the session and ask AI to pull out the highlights. Concentrate on listening, not writing things down.
4. *Give yourself the final word, even when using a modification of the Critical Response Process.* Think about how to end the discussion. You could state what new ideas the review gave you or request assistance in finding subject matter experts. Perhaps there are others in the room you want to hear from. Or maybe you would like to pose more questions of your own. Whatever you need, ensure you get it from the panel. A well-designed mock review should leave you feeling supported, energized, and clear about a way forward.

References

Heath, C., & Heath, D. (2010). *Switch: How to Change When Change is Hard*. Random House.

Lerman, L., & Borstel, J. (2003). *Critical Response Process: A Method for Getting Useful Feedback on Anything You Make, from Dance to Dessert. The Dance Exchange.*

Chapter 5
Building a Strong Foundation for Success

Almost all grant writing books and websites begin with the same advice: start early. Experienced grant writers understand that the earlier you begin the proposal-writing process, the better your final product will be. So most of us plan to do that…and then life interferes. You have competing priorities, you procrastinate, you do not receive as much help as you expected. The funding environment tightens, and you feel pressured to submit an additional proposal although you had not planned for it. A co-investigator pulls out at the last minute due to family circumstances. Your computer crashes. A tree falls on your parked car. With everything that can happen, how do you avoid running out of time?

Grant submission management has many similarities with project management. And project management is all about advance planning. Here are six principles to keep you on track and help you avoid a last-minute rush.

1. *Break everything into bite-size pieces.* Proposals usually consist of multiple components. But these might not be small enough to make your life easier. Look carefully at each task and decide whether you believe it is daunting or doable. Think of text-heavy sections, for example, as a collection of paragraphs instead of as one long chunk. To do that, outline paragraph-level content, whether as a formal outline or only as section headings. Then, concentrate on producing one paragraph at a time.

You can also break apart pieces that require less creative thinking but demand attention to detail. Collecting information about collaborators (such as biosketches or curricula vitae) is an example. This process breaks down into these tasks: acquiring all necessary documentation, making sure each document stays within the length and formatting requirements, editing for grammar and language, and, finally, looking across all documents to ensure alignment in style and information.

Avoid assuming a task is manageable without critically examining what it entails. Elements that seem easy or concise at first glance, such as creating a budget or obtaining a letter of support, may involve multistep, complicated actions. The better

C. W. Hartmann, *Grant Writing Fundamentals Made Easy*,
https://doi.org/10.1007/978-3-032-35723-6_5

you understand what your tasks entail, the more easily you can divide them into accomplishable pieces.

2. *Front-load things you lack control over.* Assess what you have control over. A final scramble over which you have control can still result in a submission. One where *other people* are in charge might result in a failure to submit. So begin with the tasks that others determine.

Make a list of what you, and only you, are responsible for. These may be important items, such as writing main parts of the text. They may also be smaller pieces, like writing an abstract or finalizing the budget. Create a timeline for completing these things that works with your schedule. (See Chap. 3, Sect. 3.3 for more on crafting reasonable timelines.)

Next, list what you must rely on others for. These are often administrative tasks (approving a budget, signing off on an application, processing forms). If others help you with the application process, these can also include final touch-ups on graphics, formatting references, or checking other documents. You may rely on experts to write various parts of the text. And letters may need to be written, sent, signed, and returned by their authors. If you require someone's help to get something done or to perfect something you drafted, do it early in your submission timeline. Be realistic. Some tasks cannot be accomplished until you have solidified what your grant will be about. But revisit your timeline frequently and adhere to the front-loading principle, even if it means interrupting the flow of your own assignments.

3. *Do distasteful things early.* When faced with difficulty, we tend to drift instead to what brings us pleasure or, at a minimum, is less arduous. This makes our present life easier but presents our future selves with problems. If you push the unpleasant parts of an application to the back burner, they will become front burner issues when you least want them there, right before submission. Anticipate and finish them earlier in the process. Space them out. Do one unpleasant task per day or per week, depending on how much time you have. Or pair tasks, one uninviting and one fun, with the fun coming last, so it acts as an incentive and reward.

But we do not always know what we do not like. I once attended a seminar where the speaker's English was translated into another language as we listened. I thought I would dislike always having to wait for the interpreter to finish. But, as it turned out, I did not mind. It slowed everything down, giving me more time to digest what I understood. During a break in the class, I spoke with the instructor, who said my reaction was common. He also explained that about once a year someone cannot tolerate the interpretation and leaves the course after only a few minutes. He smiled. "It saves time to know what you hate."

This is also true in proposal writing. If you have written applications before, you recognize the parts you find boring, annoying, or difficult. If you are new to the process, figure out what you hate by trying small portions of each task. Then allocate them according to the principles noted earlier.

4. *All hours spent on a proposal are not equal.* What is your timeframe? 2 months? 6 weeks? 10 days? Within that, how many hours can you devote to uninterrupted

work on only the proposal? And of those hours, how many are available during your times of peak productivity? Each of us has hours of the day we approach with energy and those we trudge through. Understand that you achieve more if you have more energy. Perform intellectually demanding activities in your peak times and reserve the routine, less-challenging items for your low times. Plan your proposal development process according to both the quantity and the quality of time you have. This will help you avoid the rush that arises from thinking all hours are equal.

5. *Organize tasks by size.* Inherent in these principles is the understanding that work comes in assorted sizes. You can vary the size of a task by breaking it into smaller pieces. But some will always be larger than others. So also keep track of the size of each task. On a particular day, do you only have 15 minutes between meetings? Maybe edit information about a collaborator or pull some references from the literature. On another day, when you blocked a few hours during your most productive time, tackle the significance section or work on the specific aims overview page. Altering your focus can create a sense of accomplishment and forward movement even during intervals when you have relatively little time to devote to the grant.
6. *Take your nonwork life into account.* It is tempting to think proposals will stay in their own lane, the work lane, and not creep across the line into your personal life. But early in your career or for bigger proposals, that may not be the case. Over 2 decades into my grant writing career, I routinely submit applications weeks earlier than the internal deadline. Accumulated experience, beginning the process early, and sticking to my timeline enable me to avoid rushing. But even then, life can get in the way.

The best methods for keeping a grant writing ship afloat during rough times are to (a) Build wiggle room into your timeline (see Chap. 3, Sect. 3.3), (b) Anticipate what you can, and (c) Plan for what you will do if the worst happens.

Creating extra space in your timeline enables you to absorb the shock of an unexpected family emergency, a brief illness, or snafus at work that consume more hours than desired. You are able to bounce back without panic because you know you have a cushion built in. Anticipate the stress that accompanies seasonal events (cold and flu season, major holidays) and predictable upswings in your workload. Be realistic instead of optimistic when doing this. Planning for "I might get sick" serves you better than hoping, "This will be the winter I don't get sick." Consult with colleagues and develop a strategy for dealing with common emergencies. Who will take over to push the application ahead? What can you delegate? What can you still accomplish if you cannot complete intellectually heavy tasks such as text writing? Thinking through what might happen will help you if it does. And if nothing happens, you will have more capacity to edit and otherwise refine your submission.

We have all been in situations where we had less time to finish a job than we wanted. But enacting the principles here will ensure that you never *completely* run out of time. The more you lean into advanced planning, the more your final product will reflect composure and attention to detail.

5.1 Reach out

It is dangerous to write a grant in a knowledge vacuum. You risk putting forward unsuitable ideas, making errors in the application, and wasting time and resources. But even when you have knowledge about your field and the application process, it can be challenging to determine if you have enough (and the right) information to start a proposal in the first place. In these cases, contact others before you begin.

There are three categories of people worth contacting before investing time and effort in an application. Colleagues with more experience in grant writing. Individuals who have applied for the same (or similar) opportunities. And those working for the grant-giving institution who have knowledge about the specific proposal type you hope to apply for. Whom you contact and in what order depends on your level of comfort and expertise. Even seasoned grant writers often avail themselves of all three options, because each has unique benefits.

5.1.1 Colleagues with Grant Writing and Reviewing Experience

Why do you need them? From colleagues with experience of failure, you learn what not to do. From successful colleagues, you learn how to overcome hurdles that lead to failure and techniques that lead to success. These latter individuals probably have a good grasp of their own strengths and some inkling of their own weaknesses, because they recognize that no one is a perfect proposal writer. They watch what others do and imitate what they admire. Like a good sports player, they embrace continual improvement, knowing every new application brings unexpected challenges and that each submission represents an opportunity to outdo their personal best. And colleagues who sit on grant review panels offer precious windows into the review process. This particularly benefits those early in their careers.

Successful proposal writers do not all look alike. They may be high profile or might fly under the radar. You may notice them because they continually get funded or because you stumble across one of their proposals by accident. No pattern defines who they are. What matters is that their proposals speak to you and to reviewers. Maybe you like the way the proposal hooks the reader from the first few sentences. Or that the writing is both easy to read and compelling. Perhaps the formatting of figures and tables blows you away. Or the team's accomplishments are woven throughout the narrative, unobtrusive yet convincing. No matter what the draw is, note it. Then, seek the writer out.

How to find them? If you work in an environment where your colleagues also submit grants, successful proposal writers and active reviewers may surround you. Those are fantastic circumstances. But what if you are the only grant writer at your organization, or you have been discouraged from approaching others, or everyone in your immediate environment is starting out or struggling?

In those cases, cast a wider net. If you have time and resources, attend conferences or meetings where you can meet people who write and review the types of grants you are interested in applying for. While you are there, talk about your own plans and ask for names of individuals who have prior success in similar areas. If your workplace, school, or organization has friendly ties with like-minded institutions, investigate whether those places have grant-focused seminars, workshops, or other meetings for prospective proposal writers. If they do, ask whether you may attend. Once there, treat this as a chance to network. Actively approach attendees and instructors during breaks and after sessions to talk about your plans and learn about whom you could approach for advice.

If you have none of these possibilities, use the "snowball" method. Approach one person you know or have heard of who has grant writing or reviewing experience and, after talking with them, ask whom they would speak with if they were in your shoes. Repeat this process with every person you contact, and you will soon have a list of potential contacts.

5.1.2 Individuals that Have Applied before

Why do you need them? Each grant-funding organization, large or small, has its own quirks, as do the specific calls for applications. Navigating the intricacies is easier when you have been through the process before. So if it is your first time applying, locate someone who can steer you in the right direction.

How to find the right person? If you are surrounded by individuals who have applied to similar organizations, take advantage of that wealth of knowledge. Approach experienced individuals to ask for a meeting. And if you feel as though you are alone in a grant writing desert, conduct an internet search for the name of the funding organization to which you are applying and the words "grant proposal sample." This will usually yield fruitful results, including names of those who volunteered to make their work public. You can also search for an organization's awardees from prior years. Study these people and institutions and consider which ones to approach. AI can help with this. When a search yields nothing beneficial, broaden your criteria.

> **Driver's Education for Grants**
> Think of writing a first large grant like learning how to drive a car. Yes, you can puzzle out the nuances of driving by yourself. But it is easier, faster, and safer to have an experienced individual guide you through the process. This individual does not need to drive the model of car you do. If you drive a manual transmission and learn on an automatic transmission, most aspects still apply. You can always master the quirks of a stick shift later. You learn more quickly and reach competence faster by collaborating with a person who gives advice if you panic, shares tips, and explains rules of the road.

> In proposal writing, it is possible to "tough it out" and fend for yourself. But why do that if your goal is creating the best application possible? Working with someone more experienced saves you time and frustration. You avoid common pitfalls and create more effective processes. You spend more hours crafting your argument and fewer reinventing the wheel. You use limited resources more efficiently. And all this means your ultimate product will be of higher quality. No one judges an application by whether you did everything by yourself. They judge it by what they read.

5.1.3 Individuals Who Work for the Grant-Giving Organization

Why do you need them? Someone at every organization oversees the applications that come in. It may be their full-time job or only part of what they do. Their organization may demand that they be highly trained in proposal management, or it may prefer people with diverse sets of skills. Their background matters little to you because, in the end, you want only one thing: insider knowledge.

Your job is to realize when you require that insider knowledge. You may write many successful proposals without ever contacting someone at a funding organization. But at some point, and it is frequently sooner rather than later, you will want to reach out. Or an advanced career colleague will strongly suggest it. This might be because the call for applications encourages discussion of an idea before moving too far forward. (If it does, take advantage of this open door.) You may also get in touch because your prior proposal was not funded and you would like to understand why. (Again, if this is an option, avail yourself of it.) Or you might meet a person from the organization by chance. Jump at that opportunity to discuss future funding ideas, even without a specific call for applications at hand.

How to find the right person? Look at the funding organization's website, where the information about the request for applications is housed. Also read the specific request or rejection letter, which often indicates points of contact. If you cannot discover information about any individual, call or email the department from which the money will be issued and ask with whom you could speak.

5.1.4 Setting up a Meeting

After you find an individual (successful colleague, prior applicant, or organizational representative) to contact, the next step is determining how they prefer to be approached. If you have the chance to speak with them directly (such as at a conference or during a workshop), ask them about their communication preferences. Inquire not only about the mode they usually use (email, phone, etc.) but also about the time to reach out (day of the week, hour of day). We all have moments when we are more likely to respond. Asking directly about what works best for someone increases your chance of hearing back from them. And if you do not want to ask or they cannot tell you, keep track of when they respond and when they do not and figure out their most responsive times for yourself.

If your first contact with this individual is an inquiry about a possible meeting, opt for email unless the individual (or their organization) specifically mentions a different preferred method of contact. Keep the communication brief and to the point. AI can help craft a query if you are uncertain. You only want to set up a meeting, not flood them with information. Introduce yourself. Then, follow the 1–3-2 principle (see Chap. 7, Sect. 7.1). Avoid bombarding them with facts before they say they are willing to engage with you.

Ensure it is easy for them to respond. Have one distinct "call to action," which means being clear about exactly what step you want them to take next. Proofread to check that it is only one step (e.g., "Please reply to this email with times you're available."). The more you burden them, the less likely you are to get a favorable response. Again, AI can help design a strong, clear inquiry.

5.1.5 *What to Say*

Before you contact any individual, confirm you understand your own needs. Ensure you can answer the following questions with specificity and detail. The answers to these will guide what you say when you email or speak with them.

- What is the best outcome for you regarding this exchange?
- What is your main question?
- Do you have the backup information for why you are asking that question? If you want to talk with them about a specific idea, do you have it fleshed out in enough detail to move the conversation forward? If you are interested in learning more about the current call for applications, do you have enough knowledge about it to pose clear questions? If you wish to ask more about why your proposal was not funded, what are your primary questions and why do you not know the answers yourself?
- What is the worst-case scenario for this exchange, and how will you respond if that happens?
- What is the ideal scenario for this exchange, and how will you respond if that happens?
- By the end of the exchange, what would you like the person to have done or committed to?
- What will you offer them in return?

As you learn from each person you contact, your confidence will increase. The reaching out process will become easier. And your proposal writing will improve.

5.2 Befriend Institutional Grants Administrators

I know many grants administrators. They like their jobs and are proud of their roles in helping secure and manage money for worthwhile projects. They also wish principal investigators would recognize the following.

You are not the only person I work with. Imagine having ten or more bosses, each clamoring for time and tender loving care. Your grant is significant to you. But to a grants administrator, it is one among a multitude. To them, each application may be equally important. Appreciate the obstacles these conditions impose and avoid acting like you have a right to hog the spotlight. In a grants administrator's world, only one type of principal investigator stands out from the crowd, the one who is respectful, patient, and deadline-adherent.

We are on the same team. The grants administrator's goal is the same as yours: more funding success. Administrative processes advance that goal for both of you. Each form, cutoff date, and review exists to allocate resources equitably and effectively. Accept them as necessary steps, not annoyances to be deferred or circumvented.

I may have some discretion about what I do. Think of working with grants administrators like partaking in a fine dining experience. You know the process: secure a reservation, arrive on time, be shown to your seat, peruse the menu, ask questions, order, and be served. Customers at other tables receive the same treatment. Staff are attentive but not hovering. They can also exceed expectations. Is this your first visit? Are you celebrating a special occasion? Do you need to be out the door by a certain time? Staff have no obligation to honor these extra needs. But they might choose to support you if time allows and they empathize with your situation. So when working with grants administrators, decide whether you want to be the kind of customer they sidestep or the kind for whom they go above and beyond.

My deadlines must be your deadlines. When submitting a grant, especially your first large one, the final weeks or days may be rushed. (See Chap. 3, Sect. 3.3 for tips on how to avoid this.) You may struggle to meet administrative deadlines and complete administrative tasks. But this is not the administrator's fault or responsibility. They usually shepherd many projects toward submission simultaneously. Offering one principal investigator an extension often affects how administrators can allocate resources to others. You are not a special case. You are one of many. The best strategy for managing administrative deadlines is to talk with your grants administration staff well before your submission date. Merge their timelines with yours. Accept their deadlines as your own. Believe that adhering to them helps you secure what you both want: funding.

5.3 Before Submitting a Grant

During the final days before submission, high adrenaline, nervousness, and fatigue can make you unsure of whether you did your best. Will the reviewers like it? Have you forgotten something?

Not everything is in your control. But having a punch list of things you might overlook if you do not write them down can help calm the jitters. This ensures you do not make obvious mistakes. And a clear proposal immediately shows reviewers that you care about them.

Why is this final checklist called a punch list? The phrase originates from the construction business. Contractors usually create final lists of items to correct on a project. Years ago, they wrote these lists on paper and punched holes next to completed items. Imagine the satisfaction of punching those holes and, in the end, seeing a paper riddled with them. When you create your list, I suggest you also do something memorable when you finish each task. I, for example, create my list in Excel and have a separate column entitled, "Done?" After I complete an item, I write "Yes" in the appropriate cell and highlight it a satisfying bright color. Use can different colors or shades to highlight urgent issues, indicate things in progress, and underscore items that need revisiting. Use whatever techniques work for you.

A punch list only helps if you use it. When you are tired or rushed, it can be tempting to skip part or all of the list. Resist that temptation. Ensure the checklist contains only items you will review. Think ahead about what a stressful rush feels like. Will you truly read the entire proposal again twice? Or is once already a lot to ask? Will you double-check the co-investigator biosketches for typos? Or will you assume they are fine? In other words, do not create an *ideal* punch list. Produce a *real* punch list, one with tasks that you will actually do.

No matter what you decide, a punch list involves a lot of double checking. I do not rely on my weary brain and bleary eyes for that. The computer is sharp regardless of the hour. I am not. So I use an electronic "find" function or AI to check for the following in the proposal's main documents.

- Do all references to "section" (or its equivalents) tie back to the correct section? Proposals are rarely written in order. So what was sect. A.1. may now be sect. A.3. Search for all places where you reference a different part of the proposal to ensure reviewers will look in the correct place.
- Are all placeholders for text/numbers removed? If you insert placeholders as you write, it is helpful to use things software can find, such as brackets, changes in formatting, or unusual character combinations. I use "XXX" to indicate something I plan to return to later. So I search for that.
- Is there remaining inappropriate highlighting or other formatting?

Over the course of writing a proposal, I spend almost as much time editing and reworking my one-page summary (where the specific aims or objectives are listed) as I spend on the entire rest of the proposal's narrative sections. That means I often change the wording of the aims, and sometimes even their content or scope. Because the entire final product must be consistent, I use software to discover where I mention aims throughout my other sections (including the response to reviewers document, if applicable) and ensure the wording and content is identical to the first mention (usually on the one-page aims document).

In a final review, I do (or have AI do) the following.

1. Evaluate the section heading numbers, in order. When doing this yourself, reducing the size of the manuscript to where you can see at least two pages at once helps. Reading aloud is also useful. This sounds something like, "One. One A. One A one. One A two. One B…" If numbering is out of order, I fix it.
2. I scan (or have AI scan) through all the top-level headings. Are the font style and other identifying features the same? I repeat this for the other heading levels. What I catch regularly surprises me.

I also always double-check the administrative portions of the final application, such as the first pages that contain the project number, the solicitation to which the proposal responds, and the principal investigator's name. In addition, I read the funding organization's request for applications again and make sure my submission adheres to the stated requirements. Why do I do this again at this late stage? Because it is possible to overlook mistakes. I have done that and never want to re-experience the resulting frenzy. You will have your own scares and bad experiences and will add the causes to your punch list to avoid them next time.

After I prepare my final document in the required format, I review each part. In the US, federal agencies use the Standard Form 424 format. Other funding agencies may use that or others. Doing this final check might necessitate opening attachments online or in a document. I open and check each one. Does the personnel documentation match the individuals named in the proposal (number of people included and correct names)? Do the appendices appear in the required order? Do figures and tables display correctly? I do all this even if I think, "This must be correct. I've gone over it a million times. It's stupid to check." It is *not* stupid to check. That is why it is on my punch list. The times I did not check, I overlooked errors I could have caught.

I also review the budget pages. I inspect the bottom-line numbers. Are they correct? What about the budget justification? Do the numbers there (expenses, percent effort) align with the budget? This is the last opportunity to catch inconsistencies.

The goal of a punch list is to help you avoid unreasonable flaws. Use it to eliminate all big problems and as many of the small ones as you can. And just like contractors never remove all paint splatters or buff away every nick, there is no perfect proposal. But the punch list ensures everything functions as expected, the floor plan is easy to navigate, and the first impression pops. It helps you create a house you can sell.

5.4 How to Know when you Are Ready to Submit

Knowing when a proposal is ready to submit requires experience and judgment. What happens if you do not have a lot of experience or worry about your judgment? The following are signals about submission readiness.

5.4.1 Five Signs your Proposal Is Ready to Go

1. *You started early.* As noted in many places in this book, begin the application as early as possible (see, for example, Chap. 3, Sect. 3.3). Some experts recommend a week per proposal page, meaning you may spend months putting your grant pieces together. I sometimes start a grant a year in advance. I do not work on it every day or week. But the more I contemplate, dive into the literature, and speak with colleagues, the clearer my ideas become. The times I got funded on the first try were the times I began thinking about the application early.

An advance start means several things. You understand the literature better because you have more time to search and read. You can therefore explain the relationship of your grant to the world and the need it fills. It also reduces the likelihood of making egregious errors because you build in space to review and re-review your documents. With additional time to edit, your writing is smoother. More colleagues can provide input, because you give them reasonable requests and deadlines. You pay attention to details because you are not flustered, and, therefore, items do not slip through the cracks. This results in confidence in the quality of your proposal that you will not have otherwise.

2. *Outside readers identify only minor flaws.* Enlist experienced people within or outside your field to read your proposal because their impressions will frequently mimic those of reviewers. You are often too close to the material to notice small, or even gaping, holes. Some problems may arise from this "curse of knowledge," which happens when you understand the issues so well that you fail to comprehend others do not have the same background (see Chap. 7, Sect. 7.2). Other problems can relate to a lack of attention to detail or to a faulty understanding of the existing state of the science.

It is much better to hear about any difficulties in advance than to learn about them through reviews. Outside readers view the application with fresh eyes and are not convinced of its worthiness before they pick it up. This may include readers who are not predisposed in your favor (see Chap. 4, Sect. 4.4). When outside readers suggest only minor adjustments, and you make those changes, you feel more confident about submitting.

3. *The first-page summary of the objectives (specific aims) matches the detailed plans for executing the project.* Think of the summary page as a bouillon cube

and the detailed description as soup made from that cube. In other words, this page is a condensed version of everything else in your application. This sounds easy to create. But you frequently work on this page and the rest of the text at separate times. Changes in one necessitate changes in the other. You can lose track of things or put edits off. You may set the summary page aside for a while, as you hammer out different sections of the main text. When you pick it up again, you might not notice all the places where minor changes should be made to mirror your new plans.

One technique to catch problems is to read the summary page piecemeal, jumping to each relevant section of the longer, detailed plan as it is referenced. You can also do it the opposite way, using the detailed plan as the main guide and flipping to the summary after each section. You can also enlist AI to analyze the text if you are comfortable. Whatever you do, if the documents mirror each other, pat yourself on the back. You have achieved your goal and are one step closer to being submission ready.

4. *All boxes on your tracking spreadsheet and punch list are checked.* Revisit these documents frequently during proposal preparation. I always keep track of versions of my tracking documents lists, so I know when someone last made changes. As a submission deadline approaches, it is easy to cast tracking information aside. But that is the opposite of helpful. The closer you are to submission, the more you must lean on these records. Grants can be rejected for seemingly insignificant deviations from required formatting and content. Do not let that happen to you. Keep your tracking spreadsheet and punch list detailed and updated.
5. *The final draft is not perfect, but it is in great shape.* Nothing is ever perfect. If you put away any piece of writing for a few weeks or months and revisit it, you will find things to change or maybe even errors. That happens to everyone. We have all picked up a bestseller at some point and noticed a typo. Reviewers forgive that because they make the same mistakes themselves. What reviewers are less likely to forgive is sloppiness or inattention to detail. If you feel comfortable regarding points 1–4, then your grant is likely in good shape.

Whether or not it is in *great* shape can be judged mostly by you and your colleagues. If you are unsure of your own opinion, ask someone you trust to read the proposal. Let them tell you whether you are ready to pull the trigger.

5.4.2 Five Signs you Should Wait

1. *You rushed through the application.* Proposals require constant review of minutiae. You must follow all instructions, gather necessary documentation, provide supplementary materials, and submit according to specific guidelines. Often, several pieces are not in your control. You must rely on your co-investigators

or administrators, who have their own competing demands and time constraints. Without an adequate buffer period to ensure you have adhered to all specifications, you can inadvertently miss a critical step. That alone can sink an application.

Your proposal improves with each round of polishing and editing. These rounds require time, as does pulling in the opinions of colleagues. Unless you are an experienced faculty member or researcher who can afford to submit a grant that might be rejected or reviewed unfavorably, you might not want to risk submission of an application to which you have not devoted enough resources. If you find yourself cutting corners, or even thinking about cutting corners, remind yourself that this is a danger sign of a potentially unready proposal.

2. *More experienced people have doubts.* If experienced colleagues advise waiting, listen to them, even if their input does not align with your needs or opinions. Much grant submitting wisdom comes only through practice. If people you trust, or critics you enlist, present reasonable arguments regarding why you should delay submission, pause to consider the merits of their positions.
3. *Your objectives or aims are still in flux.* Your objectives or specific aims drive your application. At the beginning of the proposal development process, you can revise them drastically, even throw ideas out in favor of better ones. You might dive deeper into the literature and realize something has been done before, or better, or there is a more compelling issue you want to address. This makes you change course. But as the application stabilizes in your mind and in the text, the scope of what you alter shrinks. Your objectives or aims solidify. Revisions are limited to wording and nuances. So if you are still making substantial changes to these components close to the submission deadline, take a step back and consider whether they will lead to success. If you are not confident, not submitting may serve you best.
4. *You see areas to improve and can afford to wait.* Without a requirement to submit your proposal, you have the luxury to decide based purely on quality. But particularly for individuals early in their careers, grants are regularly submitted in a swirl of anxiety because the trajectory of a career is at least partially tied to the funding outcome. Nevertheless, try to decide based on the merits of the application in front of you. Avoid imagining it as the application you want or hope it to be. Rather, see the application as it is. If you notice areas for improvement, or others point those out to you, fix them. The best applications are sometimes the ones that almost got submitted but were pulled at the last minute and resubmitted later.
5. *This is your first attempt at something important, and you know it is not yet the best it can be.* This situation should always give you pause. There are at least two views on how an early-stage faculty member or researcher should proceed. One camp maintains that no one can perceive in advance how reviewers will react to a specific proposal; therefore, one should simply submit it, even if it is rough, and see what happens. This is the "you never know" camp, or the "grant reviews are random" camp.

But there is another school of thought, one that maintains you are in control of a sizable portion of how reviewers react. This is the "it's not all luck" camp. Of course, any successful proposal should be based on a solid idea. It should break novel ground and address an important omission in the literature and scientific or academic knowledge base that is compelling to reviewers and funding organizations. But this camp also believes that understanding how reviewers think and crafting a proposal to maximize their cognitive ease—including careful editing and painstaking attention to writing style, details of the submission, and organization of information—helps it succeed. If you worry that reviewers will notice that you did not devote enough time to preparing an application, consider delaying.

Not everyone can afford this luxury. Sometimes you are under pressure and must submit a less than perfect product. But if you are early in your career and some of your future rides on the current application, try to uncover colleagues in the "it's not all luck" camp to support you when you propose a delay. Appreciate what motivates the individuals who want to push you into a quick submission. Often, it has something to do with money. Confer with sympathetic colleagues and mentors to devise creative solutions to any immediate funding dilemmas. Argue that by giving yourself as much time as possible, you can craft the best proposal possible and thereby increase your chance of final success.

5.4.3 When to Make the Decision

There are generally two points at which people pull a grant back. One is several weeks or months beforehand. In this case, you see the writing on the wall early. Perhaps the conundrum you wish to address is too difficult to detangle in the remaining time. You realize you require more pilot data. Or you identify a major methodological obstacle. Sometimes someone else gets funded with a similar research idea, so you need to go back to the drawing board. Or, maybe, you simply bit off more than you can chew and realize you will never finish crafting a superior product by the deadline.

The other situation happens when you are almost finished with the grant or it is only a few weeks or days before submission. Despite the progress you have made, you realize you cannot push it across the finish line without jeopardizing its chances of success. This may be because your team did not pull together the way you thought they would. Or you are still missing an essential component. Or perhaps, everyone's best efforts notwithstanding, the quality still is not as good as necessary. Whatever the reason for deciding to pull back an application instead of submitting it, try to view making that decision as its own success. The ability to recognize what does (and does not) constitute a submission-worthy application is a valuable skill. Cultivate that skill. It will serve you well.

Chapter 6
Mentored Awards for Career Development

An application for a mentored award for career development represents a unique type of submission that requires tight interweaving of multiple components. This can be the first large grant a person writes. But that does not make it the easiest. Creating a regular proposal often requires juggling at least three substantial balls: the project, the team, and the cognitive ease of the reviewer. A mentored career development award proposal, in contrast, requires juggling at least five: the applicant, the project, the mentoring team, the training plan, and the cognitive ease of the reviewer.

6.1 Mentors

A mentor can protect, promote, and propel your career. Having at least one person willing to step into the proposal thinking and writing fray makes applications easier to write and, generally, increases the likelihood of success. Anyone can use a good mentor. But individuals early in their careers rely on them more, particularly when submitting mentored award applications.

There are two paradigms in which mentorship may operate.

I call the paradigm of individual effort in a vacuum the "sink-or-swim" paradigm. This type of mentoring may seem fantastic on paper and can be insidiously destructive in its operationalization. It usually looks like this. An early career person pairs with a mentor who has excellent credentials in their field. The surrounding environment may have many other strong scholars in this discipline. The institution and those who operate within it set high expectations, which feels exciting. And the entire system operates with an unexpressed understanding that a talented early career individual will rise to the top regardless of the amount of support they receive. The (incorrect but firmly implied) logic is that talent drives success and failure results primarily from lack of talent. Often, these environments intimate (but may not say directly) that *less*

C. W. Hartmann, *Grant Writing Fundamentals Made Easy*,
https://doi.org/10.1007/978-3-032-35723-6_6

mentoring is better because a trial by fire will separate the Olympic swimmers from the dog paddlers. Self-sufficiency of the early career person reigns supreme.

In these environments, mentoring is conspicuous for its absence. The institution and all associated with it assume any failure to receive a mentored award is the fault of the applicant and not due to lack of support. Sinking instead of swimming proves what was always there to be proven: that the individual was "not good enough" to succeed.

Environments like this churn through early career folks because they think of them as plentiful and expendable. Those who finally emerge as Olympic swimmers tend to accept that a solitary journey was inevitable, even valuable. That is understandable. In the sink-or-swim paradigm, the long and painful process of attempting to succeed without help is the right one. Assistance lessens the sweetness of the final victory. Doing it on your own is the highest achievable goal.

But that, frankly, is baloney. Mentoring is not a crutch. In the directly opposed "support-and-collaboration" paradigm, good mentoring is a wind beneath a person's wings, or, to continue the prior analogy, a current that helps propel a swimmer in their chosen direction. Individuals swimming without a current will never know how much faster and farther they would have gone with a supportive one.

For early career faculty and researchers, finding the right current, the right mentor, is key. This should be a mentor who espouses support and collaboration as worthy goals. Working with this type of mentor should propel a career. It is also important to recognize that treading water where you *thought* there was a current is a signal to try elsewhere. You may be your own worst enemy if part of you believes failure to progress is a sign of weakness. Bring this reaction to the surface for critical appraisal. Is this what *you* believe? Or are you responding to what your past or present environment suggests is true?

The following is a four-step survival guide for those early in their careers aiming to submit mentored awards. Whether you are in academia, industry, the nonprofit world, or government, you need good mentoring within the appropriate mentoring paradigm to support you in swimming as fast and far as you can. If you already have good mentoring, the tips here may improve your situation. If you are not sure what type of mentoring environment you are in, look at what surrounds you. If you notice signs of the sink-or-swim paradigm and you buy into self-sufficiency at all costs, recognize your role in that paradigm and take active steps, such as those here, to extract yourself.

6.1.1 Step 1: Recognize Good Mentoring

Good mentors do not all look the same. Some are relatively hands off. Others are more engaged. But they all share basic characteristics.

They are available when you need them. You may have to adjust yourself to their style, and they to yours. The primary mentor on my own mentored early career award never scheduled meetings with me. But he had an open-door policy. When I knocked on his door (literally or virtually), he would either meet with me immediately or tell me when to come back that day. He also took time to give meaningful, detailed feedback on my manuscripts, proposals, and grant execution. In the ways that counted, he was always there when I needed him.

Good mentors make time for you. They participate in writing and review drafts before you show them to the rest of the world and help you understand your field's explicit and implicit rules and how to refine your work. They smooth the path you want to walk. Your relationship with them is a collaboration, not an assignment.

They put your needs above their own. Watch whether your mentor continually takes credit for your results, demands to be first author on papers or principal investigator on grants, is always the public speaker, or closes the door on conversations that would benefit you. These are signs of bad mentoring. A good mentor sees a mentee's career path as distinct from their own. They value and foster conversations about a mentee's goals and plans. If a conflict in direction arises, they support the mentee. By definition, a mentor is at a more advanced career stage. They should not need to squash a mentee's career to grow their own. Yes, their collaboration with you builds their own curriculum vitae. But altruism, not personal advancement, should primarily drive their interactions, particularly around your proposal.

Near the start of my professional journey, I chose to extract myself from a bad mentoring relationship, something many people were angry with me about. But my primary mentor backed me up. He argued my case at the highest levels, calmly and without drama, even though it exposed him to criticism. He probably would not have made the same choice as I did, had he been in my shoes. Yet he trusted that my decision was right for me and never wavered in his support.

They are open to constructive observations. In a long-term relationship such as mentoring, people will inevitably step on each other's toes. When your mentor crosses a line, intentionally or not, you may want to speak up. (AI can dig into the peer-reviewed literature on communication, diagram conversations based on scientific evidence, and role-play them with you.) How your mentor reacts to feedback will teach you a lot about who they are and whether you are a decent fit. A good mentor is open to professional discussions about boundaries, relationships, and what matters to a mentee.

They do not play favorites or triangulate. One of the last things you want is a mentor who fosters a cut-throat, gossipy, or distrustful environment. It may feel terrific to be the current favorite. But someone who plays favorites has unclear motivations. Your proposal will benefit more from honest collaboration and positive team building.

They do not operate only in a small, exclusive circle. Identify whether and how your mentor collaborates. A good mentor works well with others. These may be colleagues you like and, at least, should be individuals who appreciate and respect each other's strengths. Keep your ears pricked for hints of an "us vs. them" mentality. While success in academia is frequently equated with competition, good mentors avoid fierce struggles within their own teams. Us vs. them equates with a scarcity mindset. At some point, your mentor could decide you (and your mentored award) are no longer "us" and are no longer worthy of resource investment. That decision is out of your control. The relationship is not.

You feel safe. There is a strong literature base regarding the importance of psychological safety for creating successful teams, as described by Amy Edmondson in *The Fearless Organization: Creating Psychological Safety in the Workplace for Learning, Innovation, and Growth* (2018). A mentoring relationship is intimate. Mentors may see you struggle. You might expose your own weak points in front of them. To collaborate effectively on a mentored award, you need security. If you do not have it, you will avoid sharing drafts and speaking frankly about your ideas. Your proposal will suffer.

6.1.2 Step 2: Help your Mentor Improve

A resource for developing or improving mentor–mentee relationships is an individual development plan. These plans are often used for postdoctoral students and can be tweaked to apply to any situation. There are many examples online to choose from. You can enlist AI to refine one to fit your circumstances. As you do, think about the support-and-collaboration paradigm and what support you require for a mentored award application. Bring your draft plan to your mentor. Talk about specifics. Discuss how having a plan in place holds both of you accountable.

6.1.3 Step 3: Find Other Mentors

You do not need only one mentor. Mentored awards for career development almost always require a mentoring team. A mentor operating within the support-and-collaboration paradigm will be open to your finding other mentors and may even assist you in doing so. If your primary mentor does not believe in that paradigm, finding other mentors who do may save your application. Additional mentors can be at distant locations. You may never meet face-to-face. They may mentor you in only one subject. Good mentoring comes in all shapes and sizes but will always create an environment that helps you draw satisfaction and self-esteem from the collaborative effort.

6.1.4 Step 4: Recognize that you May be Part of the Problem

Of the two mentoring paradigms, sink-or-swim may be the more prevalent. It is certainly more difficult to recognize, both within yourself and within others, because it evokes pressure to prioritize self-reliance and independence. This seems worthy. But complete self-sufficiency in academia and the research world is an illusion. No one succeeds alone, no matter what they believe. Mentored award applications suffer when people early in their careers write them unassisted.

In the support-and-collaboration paradigm, you learn that prioritizing support and collaboration helps uncover strengths. This increases your capabilities and sense of self-worth. So dissect your own beliefs thoroughly. Expose remnants of the sink-or-swim paradigm and embrace them only if you—not the world in which you live—think they serve you and your proposal best.

6.2 Peer Mentoring for Award Writing

A mentor at a more advanced career stage can leverage their knowledge, networks, and funding to your advantage. But it is also possible, even desirable, to create peer mentor networks of fellow academics or researchers at your own level. For the difficult and important task of writing a mentored award for career development, peer mentoring can serve many functions.

It provides support. A mentored award application requires a lot of work, much of it in unfamiliar territory. You negotiate new regulations and requirements in a high-stakes environment. If you are isolated, you may constantly reinvent the wheel. If, on the other hand, you create a peer network of one or more individuals also applying, you can split tasks, provide comments on drafts, and share different approaches and templates. Working together to mentor each other enables greater insight than one person can achieve alone. Potentially, it also directly or indirectly facilitates input from other people's formal mentoring teams.

Peer mentoring can fill gaps. Your current mentoring relationships may be rocky or absent. Or your proposal may branch into fields outside your current mentors' areas of expertise. In these cases, peer mentorship may provide powerful support. (Ideally, your existing mentors will introduce you to peers, but not everyone works in an ideal world.) For mentors who feel unsettled by the inclusion of additional specialists, peer mentorship often flies safely under the radar. Find colleagues at your level who have expertise outside your own or experiences to draw on.

Peer mentoring can promote accountability. We all have moments where we want to ditch our sensible plans for writing and procrastinate. Having at least one peer to whom we feel accountable can enable us to meet deadlines we might otherwise ignore because it is usually easier to send an incomplete or early draft to a peer. It can also be easier to hear their honest feedback and listen to them when they remind you of your original plans.

Peer mentoring can boost your productivity. Whether you have problems setting and adhering to deadlines or your publication record needs a lift before you submit your application, peer mentoring groups may help. You can, for example, create a writing team that tackles a series of papers where each of you is first author at least once. You can organize peer reviews for grant submissions, create timelines together, and engage each other's work from fresh perspectives. You may also benefit from a writing accountability model. You may, for example, sit together, virtually or in person, at a specific time every week to write, whether it is on the same project or different ones. Being in a room with other people who are also writing motivates progress.

Whatever form your peer mentoring group takes, create it with the same consideration you give to choosing a more advanced career mentor. Ensure you feel safe with the members of your group, that they are people you respect and enjoy spending time with. Make sure the group meets your needs and those of others involved. You can collaborate for the duration of a single application or may meet for many years. The group can be small or large. It may always have only the same members or shrink and grow over time. Your needs dictate what you do, because peer mentoring groups have only one purpose: to support you in becoming the person you want to be.

6.3 Intertwining all Components of a Mentored Award Application

Mentored grant applications for early career development frequently take more time to write because, as indicated already, they necessitate more intricate alignment of their multiple components than many equivalent-sized applications do. Most instructions for these types of awards require information about four different components: the proposed project, the applicant's career to date and goals for the future, the mentors involved, and the training that will take place during the award period. These must all relate to each other. In other words, from the beginning stages of the grant writing process, applicants and their teams need to think about a coherent thread that supports reviewers' cognitive ease, a thread reviewers can follow and find compelling. Here is an example.

Imagine an applicant, Kai, who has a bachelor's degree in history, a master's degree in psychology, and a PhD in public health. Kai is now in the final year of a postdoctoral fellowship in cancer epidemiology. He wants to apply for a mentored award from an organization focused on health systems research. Only looking at his degrees and training thus far, Kai's career has not been a straight line. One task, therefore, is to decide on a story about why he is the right candidate.

Just as there is no perfect writing, there is no perfect story. In mentored awards, it is dangerous to cement a career story without considering the other parts of the proposal, such as the project and the training plan. Still, beginning the process involves finding connections among Kai's career path milestones. In this imaginary case, it could be cancer. Let us imagine Kai worked after college for two years as a marketing materials developer at a startup biotech company that happened to focus on cancer drugs. What he learned there about cancer and its effects on patients' psychological health led to the master's degree in psychology. During that program, his thesis advisor organized a volunteer excursion to set up a mental health clinic in an oncology department in a foreign hospital. Kai joined the trip. What he saw ignited a passion for public health, in which he received a PhD. Then, he chose his postdoctoral position because he wanted to supplement his doctoral program's basic instruction in epidemiology and statistics with additional advanced training and opportunities to participate in research studies. Only one of the studies he worked on during the postdoctoral program focused on cancer. But if Kai's mentored award project centers on cancer, this can become the backbone of a career story.

To be clear, most people notice a common thread that ties together their education and career *after* the fact. Imaginary Kai probably did not begin college with his eyes set on cancer. But it represents a possible narrative. A mentored award does not need to describe every tangent in a person's path. It needs to describe a linked journey. Constructing this may feel artificial. You may bristle at the idea of leaving out important aspects of your life. But you must present a clear and logical larger picture for *the reviewer*. They need to see how *parts* of your history (not *every* part) lead to the work proposed.

Kai and his team will also decide which gaps in his education and training the award will fill and how those relate to the proposed project. Taking more epidemiology coursework would, of course, lack plausible justification. But if the project involved interviews with patients or clinicians working in a healthcare system, and if Kai's education on how to conduct research interviews and analyze the resulting data was limited, then studying qualitative methods during the award (before he needs them for the project) would likely make sense to reviewers.

And in the intricate web of mentored award applications, if Kai proposed conducting interviews in the project and proposed training on qualitative methods, he would also require an expert in qualitative methods on the mentoring team. Depending on Kai's prior experience and the dominance of interviews in the project, this mentor might not need to be heavily involved. But Kai would certainly benefit from someone advising on the project.

Another person Kai would probably need on the mentoring team is someone with expertise in the clinical aspects of cancer care since Kai is not a clinician. This then leads to the question of whether the training plan might benefit from, for example, Kai's shadowing a clinician in a cancer clinic. How much training and mentoring is available in this regard may, in turn, affect the project's research questions and design.

These types of awards also walk a thin line between giving the applicant enough support to succeed and not reproducing the careers of the mentors. The goal of these awards is to create *independence*. If Kai's application mirrors the work of his mentors too closely, reviewers may question the mentors' motives and Kai's likelihood of launching his own career.

In addition, any project is always developed and justified in relationship to existing knowledge. But you cannot propose a project *only* because there is a gap in the literature (see Chap. 3, Sect. 3.2). Reviewers must understand the project's background and how the candidate's experiences match with the area of interest.

It is also difficult to convince reviewers without data. Yet Kai does not have much prior work in his chosen area to reference. Viable solutions include Kai's using existing databases to gather compelling information, competing for a small award before the mentored award to collect his own pilot data, or collaborating with mentors who have pilot data on which he can build his own line of research. Each of these options also has ramifications for various components of the submission.

Kai's example highlights how these types of applications involve complex juggling to create an overarching story that reviewers find compelling and easy to believe. Reviewers for these applications must understand substantial information about different subjects at once. The clearer the narrative, and the more visible and convincing the components by which they will judge the proposal and advocate for it in a review committee meeting, the easier their job.

Reference

Edmondson, A. (2018). *The Fearless Organization: Creating Psychological Safety in the Workplace for Learning, Innovation, and Growth.* Wiley.

Chapter 7
Techniques to Enable Cognitive Ease

Have you ever read a book and lost track of time? I remember reading one of my favorite books in a modern pizza café in Kathmandu in 1986 (the *only* modern pizza café in Kathmandu in 1986). I sat alone with my lunch in the blue-tiled room, on a stool by the front window, unable to stop flipping pages. Hours passed. When I finally looked up, the sun was setting over the Himalayas.

Chances are, you have experienced something similar. You forgot you were reading words on a page and simply "heard" the words as though they were spoken to you. All other awareness faded. In that ideal reading state, time stopped. A magical stream of sentences carried you forward.

Cognitive ease plays an influential role in that sensation (for more on cognitive ease, see Chap. 1, Sect. 1.1). Cognitive ease lessens a reader's cognitive load and decreases the burden on working memory. It creates a feeling that reading is effortless, the people who wrote the text are good, the information is familiar, and the arguments are true. It exists in relation to its counterpart, cognitive strain, which increases cognitive load and overwhelms working memory, demanding significant mental effort. Daniel Kahneman describes both in detail in his book *Thinking, Fast and Slow* (2011). To illustrate the concept, Kahneman suggests thinking of cognitive ease and strain as two opposite points on a dial. At full strain, any sense of ease evaporates. At zero strain, the brain feels no need for exertion.

In our daily lives, we cycle unconsciously from ease to strain and back again. Rereading a sentence because of a typo or difficult grammatical structure causes strain. We glide back into ease when sentences are short and well written. If we squint to see the tiny-print results of an online survey on a smartphone, we induce strain. On the phone, expanding the text to enlarge the numbers enables our brain to relax back into ease.

You may be proficient at writing and an expert in your subject area. But if you do not understand how a proposal interacts with a reader, you are missing a key that influences the review process. A strong application enables a reviewer to ignore distractions. The text, graphics, and layout create a cognitive experience that promotes

C. W. Hartmann, *Grant Writing Fundamentals Made Easy*,
https://doi.org/10.1007/978-3-032-35723-6_7

ease. Deep immersion in ease allows the reviewer to see only what is directly in front of them. External noise and outside visual stimuli fade. Their mind focuses on the proposal.

Specific techniques foster the circumstances that make this possible. This chapter introduces the most important techniques, with examples and exercises.

7.1 Employ the 1–3-2 Principle

These days, marketing solicitations and newsletters crowd email inboxes. Large companies employ teams of professionals and AI to compose, edit, and assess every sentence. But smaller firms lack this infrastructure, sometimes resulting in less polished text. Here, for example, is a fictional email from a local farm stand. As you read, take note of what you think are the most important pieces of information.

"It's spring! If you're like us, by January you were already sick of the snow and itching to get back into the garden. Unfortunately, the sudden low temperatures two weeks ago wiped out some early crops. But the good news is that other plants are growing and the farm stand is now open. The frigid winter also took its toll on our driveway. Potholes abound. We will have the driveway paved next Tuesday and Wednesday. When that happens, we will close the stand for a few hours. Right now, we have a nice variety of veggies."

What main points did you gather from the message? Where are they located?

Exercise: Rewrite the Marketing Email

Rewrite the farm stand email, using the existing phrasing as much as you like. Reorder sentences or write new ones. Jot down the updated version or say it aloud. Do *not* use AI. Take only a few minutes for this exercise.

Wait to read further until you are finished.

What crossed your mind as you reordered the paragraph? Why did you make the choices you made? Did you consult with your own sense of cognitive ease while you edited?

Likely, you noticed these two points in the original email: that the farm stand is now open and that it will be closed parts of Tuesday and Wednesday. Where did you put this information in your revision?

A primary strategy for prioritizing cognitive ease is the 1–3-2 principle (which can also be the 2–3-1 principle). The principle, in either case, means you bury the least important material in the middle and lead and finish with the important pieces. Put the *essential* element either first or last, your choice. I learned of this principle in Roy Peter Clark's *Writing Tools: 50 Essential Strategies for Every Writer* (2008), the book I recommend most often for those who want to learn to edit. The principle applies at all levels of a proposal or any other text: sentence, paragraph, summary, and entire document. I find it the single most effective technique for improving a reader's cognitive ease.

One foundation for this principle is that English speakers remember what comes first. This is driven by standard English conventions. In English, the initial words and phrases of any piece of writing usually serve as orienting tools. Read these two sentences quickly aloud.

Sentence A: Whether or not our partner institutions support this initiative, our organization intends to invest resources.

Sentence B: Our organization intends to invest resources in this initiative, whether or not our partner institutions support it.

Which was easier to comprehend?

In both sentences, the key point is that "our organization intends to invest resources." Sentence A leaves it until the end, making a reader plow through a long introduction. Sentence B puts it up front. Sentence B is thus easier to understand.

At the sentence level, think of the subject and verb of a sentence as coat hangers. The rest of the information is clothing. You strain readers less when you give them the coat hangers early and do not require them to hold an armful of clothes while waiting for a way to organize them.

At the paragraph or section level, a proposal writer can guide a reader by consistently placing an overview or instructive heading first, making subsequent details easier to understand. Because reviewers are often short on time, they may need to skim parts. Or they may read the application quickly, looking for specific subject matter as they review. The principle of keeping critical information first enables any reader to find and digest content quickly, promoting ease.

Why should important messages come last? In *Thinking, Fast and Slow* (2011), Kahneman describes numerous research experiments that consistently show that we are most likely to remember (1) the most intense moments and (2) endings of experiences. We also judge an entire experience based mostly on our assessment of those two components. This is the "peak-end rule" of remembering and evaluating.

To illustrate the rule, Kahneman describes a study of colonoscopies from the 1990s, before the widespread use of anesthetic and amnesic drugs. Researchers prompted many patients to assess their pain level during colonoscopies every 60 seconds on a scale of zero (no pain at all) to ten (intolerable pain). Researchers also asked the patients to give the entire event an overall rating. As an example, Patient A had a relatively short procedure, and Patient B's procedure was more than twice as long. Otherwise, the two patients had similar experiences. During their procedures, both patients' pain ratings went up and down. Both had the same rating for their worst pain, an eight. But just before the end of their procedures, Patient A gave a final rating of seven, and Patient B gave a final rating of one. In other words, Patient A's experience was short but ended painfully. Patient B's was long but ended without pain.

From the researchers' perspective, both patients had the same "peak" experience of pain, meaning they rated their worst moment the same. They both experienced intermittent pain. But Patient A spent considerably less time in pain because the procedure was much shorter. Thus, from a moment-to-moment perspective, you would want to be Patient A. But when researchers compared how the two patients *remembered* their experiences through their overall ratings, Patient B, who ended without pain, gave the experience a much better overall pain rating than Patient A.

This is the peak-end rule in action. The duration of the experience did *not* play into these patients' overall ratings. Researchers believe our memory of an experience is predicted by the most intense moment (which was the same for both Patient A and B) and by how it ended (B's ended much better than A's). So while you may want to be A as you go through the colonoscopy, you want to be B when you remember it.

Of course, reading a grant should have little in common with undergoing a colonoscopy. The connection between the two exists in the importance of understanding that it is the person undergoing the event, not anyone else, who gives the final judgment of how the experience was for them. For colonoscopies, the evaluation is given by a patient, for proposals, by a reviewer.

In grant writing, the peak-end rule underscores the significance of (1) creating powerful moments that engage a reviewer's emotions and (2) positioning valuable information last. In practice, the rule stresses the potential value of inserting a meaningful story or anecdote to produce a peak moment. It also highlights the significance of strategically crafting memorable endings for key sections and for the application as a whole.

How do you know what is most important (the 1 and 2 positions in 1–3-2 or 2–3-1)? The urge to bold, underline, or otherwise highlight text in the middle of something is perhaps the strongest clue. If you find yourself bolding a phrase in the center of a sentence or calling out the second paragraph in a three-paragraph section, stop. Analyze why you did this. People do not remember text simply because it has a different font style. They remember first, peak, and last. So instead of bolding a middle item, reorganize. Move the information to the first or last position, whichever makes the most sense. The proposal writing and editing process involves critically appraising all text from this perspective. Let the priority of your content drive how you present information.

Where is this principle most neglected? In an application's initial summary or overview. How to best summarize an application is covered in Chap. 10. But in brief, lead with your main point, couched in a compelling sentence. Then, look at all paragraphs or sections in the summary. Does each begin and end with its most important ideas? Do you create a peak experience for the reader, a moment where you engage their emotions or challenge them with a compelling question? Do you bold, underline, or italicize middle text? Reorder sentences or split paragraphs until what counts comes first and last. Next, examine the overall structure. Does the first paragraph engage and convince? Does the final paragraph conclude with a bang, a take home message that makes the reviewer nod and think, "Yes, we should fund this"?

Of course, this principle also applies at the level of the entire proposal. Do you start with a hook? (For more on hooks, see Chap. 9.) If the instructions tell you to end the main narrative with a project or study team management plan, do you construct a memorable finish by linking that plan to a final sentence or paragraph that ties your entire application into an impressive, must-fund bundle?

When you feel comfortable applying the principle, you will discover myriad opportunities to practice, even in emails and text messages. How often have you hunted through someone's email to find the point? Let others benefit from your commitment to increasing cognitive ease.

Make the 1–3-2/2–3-1 principle part of your daily routine, like remembering to brush your teeth twice a day or stretch every hour. As you integrate it, you will become aware of more places to apply it. That practice will help you organize and edit your next grant.

7.2 Combat the Curse of Knowledge

You write a proposal for reviewers. Not to wow them with how much you know. But to impress them with your argument. They should finish the application thinking, "I get that, we need that, and these people are the right ones to do that." The last thing you want is a reviewer who thinks, "What the heck was that about? I couldn't understand a thing."

But all writers face a hurdle described by Chip and Dan Heath in their book *Made to Stick: Why Some Ideas Survive and Others Die* (2007): the difficulty of understanding the perspective of someone who does not have the same information as you. The Heath brothers call it "the curse of knowledge." It affects everyone who has any subject matter expertise in anything.

My spouse, Ron, is among the most experienced long-distance hikers in the nation. He began hiking seriously approximately 60 years ago. His backpacking knowledge has filled books. When Ron took me, a complete novice, for my first serious, multiday backpacking adventure, he knew he had to dumb it down.

Ron ran his initial plan by his hiking buddies, who told him that the arrangement was too ambitious. He modified it. They okay-ed the revision. So did I. It sounded beautiful. I thought I could do it. After all, for someone with a desk job, I was in decent shape. And I wanted to experience part of his world.

For the hike, a friend dropped us off in what someone later described as "one of the most isolated parts of the Lower Forty-eight." That was the start of a 100-mile hike on a poorly marked trail. My misery began a few minutes after we watched his friend's pickup disappear in a cloud of dust kicked up by wild cattle. The scrappy trail petered out. Ron pointed at a mountain in the distance. "Not a problem. I know where we're going. We just need to hike over there."

We stomped through thigh-high brush, along thin animal trails, and across precarious ridges. The scenery's drama, colors, distances, and light astonished me. But physical discomfort elbowed its way into every minute I was not sitting down. I developed blisters. I could not keep up. I had visions of one of us breaking a leg and the other walking for days to get help. I will spare you more details and only say that the hike ended 50 miles early, thanks to cell phone reception at the top of a peak. The best part of the adventure for me was when a different buddy of his arrived in his van at a trail head to pick us up.

Later, Ron and I analyzed what went wrong. He had tried to create a memorable and fun adventure. He had consulted with other experts. He wanted me to like backpacking, not hate it. But he was too advanced in the field to remember what a novice did not know. So he forgot to coach me on what he already understood. We decided what we would do differently if we ever did it again. Instead of my hopping on an elliptical machine in my basement a few times a week, Ron would take me for practice hikes on real trails in real woods. I would strap on a loaded backpack and my hiking shoes when I walked to the grocery store. And we would watch YouTube videos about the proposed section of trail, so I would not be surprised by its isolation. In other words, we would actively combat Ron's curse of knowledge.

In the grant world, reviewers are me. Proposal writers are Ron. Writers want to showcase the best of their world and design an unforgettable experience. But they are not novices and cannot easily see their world from an outsider's eyes. Yet the curse of knowledge means they will *think* their explanations are easy to understand and will skip over crucial details because they *think* everyone else knows them or, worse yet, because they do not notice that they forgot to include them.

The curse of knowledge is a *curse* because it blinds you to what you need to be aware of. When suffering from it, writers inadvertently create cognitive strain for readers.

In proposal writing, one strategy for overcoming this issue is to translate ideas into concrete language. Use imagery that relates the idea to something outside your field. Do not be afraid of simplifying while maintaining accuracy. Employ words that refer to tangible demonstrations of how things work. Draw analogies. The more complex your main idea, the more valuable imagery, analogy, or simplification is in providing a scaffold onto which an outsider can grasp.

Most of us, for example, cannot easily fathom the complexities of the research that lies behind recommendations about whether to obtain routine screening for various types of cancer. So experts devised a simple analogy to help people understand what type of cancer may benefit most from screening. This is known as the turtle, bird, rabbit analogy.

Imagine a turtle, a bird, and a rabbit in a barn, all trying to escape. Each animal represents a type of cancer. Screening enables you to open the barn door a crack to see the animal (see that you have cancer) and take steps to secure the barn to prevent the animal from escaping (prevent death). But the lethargic, plodding turtle will never escape the barn in the first place. It is analogous to a slow growing cancer. People die *with* turtle cancer, not *from* it. Birds are different. Whether or not you open the door, the bird will escape out of a window. This is analogous to an aggressive cancer for which there is no curative treatment. Even if it is detected early, this cancer is invariably fatal. Rabbit cancers are yet a third type: they can be trapped in the barn if they are noticed early enough, before they have burrowed a tunnel out. If detected early, this cancer is treatable. Screenings are most valuable if they detect rabbit cancers for which there are viable treatment options. This simple but accurate analogy orients non-clinicians to the key issues. In a grant about cancer screening, a writer using this analogy could follow with more specifics.

Another technique for averting the problems that arise from the curse of knowledge is to ask people completely outside your field to read your proposal. Invite their constructive criticism. Even busy individuals will sometimes volunteer to examine a paragraph or two. They will see what you cannot. Ask them to be honest about where they stumble. Chapter 4, Sect. 4.4 describes the types of people whose perspectives can be helpful and Chap. 4, Sect. 4.5 gives guidance on how to have productive dialogues with them.

The curse plagues everyone. The cure is to identify its effects and treat them.

7.3 Avoid Jargon

Jargon is related to the curse of knowledge. Jargon is insider shorthand, a specialized vocabulary for members of a specific field. It helps these specialists communicate with each other with precision, accuracy, and rapidity. But jargon means little to others, including reviewers who come from outside a particular area. What counts as jargon may be difficult for you to identify because you are, yourself, an insider. So learn to identify field-specific terms. Then cultivate the flexibility to describe your own area without resorting to jargon.

Exercise: Working with Jargon

The Alda Center for Communicating Science conducts workshops where participants take part in the following exercise. The more you adhere to the instructions, the more benefit you will gain from the experience. Do each step in the order written, finishing one before proceeding to the next. Do not read ahead.

1. *Write down (on a computer, mobile device, or piece of paper) five keywords that describe your specific area of expertise.* Choose your terms as though you were doing it for a scholarly or professional audience. If you work in multiple areas, choose one. Spend only a minute or two on this. Select the key terms that come to mind, the ones that describe your area accurately. Be honest.
2. *Find a listener.* This can be any adult, even a stranger, anyone who is willing to listen to you for about a minute. Stop reading these instructions until you have found that listener.

   STOP HERE UNTIL YOU HAVE A LISTENER.
3. *Show the listener your five keywords.*
4. *Have the listener time you.* You have 1 min.
5. *Now, explain your area of expertise without using any of the keywords.* That is right. You must avoid using any keywords. Instruct your listener to stop you if you do. And if you do, you have to start over.
6. *Go!*
7. *After you finish, ask your listener how easy it was for them to understand what you said.*

When I attended a workshop, over one hundred scientists did this exercise. Everyone found it difficult to do but a pleasure to listen to. Speakers felt like they were twisting themselves into pretzels to avoid saying the keywords. But listeners found the explanations clear.

My breakout group consisted of three other scientists: a computational chemist, a positive psychologist, and an expert on the internet. None of us was familiar with the content of what anyone else did. All of us left the exercise understanding each other's subjects better. When I explained my area of expertise, my explanation felt circuitous and long-winded. Yet my listener found what I said interesting, even compelling. It showed me the seemingly impossible task was not only possible but also helpful.

The exercise asks you not to read ahead, because once you know the point of the exercise, the temptation is to pick keywords you can easily avoid. When applying this technique to a proposal, choose jargon from something you or your organization has written. Stick with those. Then, rework your text to describe your message without using jargon.

Reviewers will not necessarily come from your field. Often, you are lucky to have one person on a review panel whose expertise aligns with yours. So it pays to strengthen the muscles that enable you to express yourself without jargon. The more ease reviewers feel as they read explanations and arguments, the better they will understand your work.

7.4 Be Consistent

Consistent use of terminology and ordering of concepts sounds easy to do. It might be if you wrote the entire text of an application in one fell swoop. But I have yet to encounter anybody who does that. Grants are usually written piece-by-piece, often not in the final order the reviewer sees. That is how problems creep in. Inconsistency causes cognitive strain and, in the worst case, can jeopardize a reviewer's understanding of a proposal's arguments.

Inconsistent use of terminology is an easy trap to fall into. Imagine your application is about ocean wildlife. Throughout the proposal you might, deliberately or inadvertently, employ many different terms to describe this: marine life, aquatic creatures, sea life, or ocean creatures. This may feel appropriate, because at some point you learned repetition is bad, that you should "vary your wording." But scientific writing benefits, above all, from clarity. Clarity is achieved by defining terms on first use and consistently employing the same terms to refer to the same phenomena. Even slight changes in wording, such as switching randomly between the terms marine life, ocean life, and sea life, can suggest ambiguity about the topic of investigation.

A reviewer often reads or skims an application in the order of the final product. This means that if you state in the brief summary, which usually appears first, that your grant is about turtles, dolphins, and whales, reviewers absorb those concepts in that order. Confusion arises if the subsequent one-page overview then discusses dolphins, whales, and turtles, and the following narrative sections describe the importance of whales, turtles, and dolphins. This may feel like a minor issue for someone fully familiar with all the concepts introduced. But you cannot count on a reviewer being as acquainted with your subject as you are. And even an expert appreciates a cognitively easy experience. Pick a phrase and an order for your concepts and stick to those from first to last.

7.5 Show, Don't Tell

A proposal writer generally operates under strict page limits. To save space, it is tempting to summarize points, opting for vague brevity instead of supporting each component with concrete descriptions. Here is why that is a bad idea and what to do instead.

General statements do not convince. Which contractor would you hire, the one who says, "I have a lot of satisfied customers" or the one who says, "Here's a portfolio of my recently finished projects, including photographs, timelines, and testimonials"? You may think you save space and time by condensing your points. But when you are vague or general, you raise questions in reviewers' minds. They wonder about the strength of the foundation for the points you make and may assume they have less support than they do. You may raise suspicions that you are glossing over something or sweeping issues under the rug. Reviewers do not want to read that a problem is "critical" (telling). They want to read about the "50,000 people diagnosed every week" (showing).

You may feel words such as "uniquely," "importantly," "groundbreaking," or "transformative" will stealthily direct a reviewer to think like you do. But buzzwords rarely work as intended and may even annoy. Try replacing them with specific information, using phrases such as, "a replicated finding that overturned older studies' results" or "based on pilot data, we developed a new theory." Reviewers do not believe or remember things simply because you tell them to. They believe and remember because you convince them.

Aligned with this principle is presenting a compelling answer to the, "So what?" question, meaning answering why a reviewer and funding organization should care about the proposal's main issues. Imagine your reader has a big "convince me" button on their head that you need to push repeatedly with the most effective tools possible. Ideally, every sentence in your text should relate clearly to that button. Key sentences must push it hard. By the time the reader finishes the application, they should be convinced.

General statements are not memorable. How many times have you heard or read a statement like the following, "This research will impact XYZ"? That may sound good to the person who wrote it. But your reviewers will remember your messages better if you give examples, the more specific and novel, the better. Explain your points with precision, using statistics, data, or citations. Instead of "major improvement," say there was a "42% increase," or you "replicated the finding in two other populations," or "the intervention has been adopted by five industry leaders." Delete, "Our intervention is highly effective," and replace it with, "After implementation of our intervention across four hospitals, procedure completion rates rose from 53% to 79%."

Examples answer questions before they are asked. Anticipate concerns instead of raising them. Avoid creating logic holes and gray areas. Flesh out the reasons behind your points. If your explanations are thorough, a reviewer will nod and move on.

Examples can tell a story. If you want to be creative, weave your examples into a story. An anecdote might be as short as one sentence. Give reviewers a picture that sticks in their minds. If you need inspiration, Chip and Dan Heath devote their book *Made to Stick: Why Some Ideas Survive and Others Die* (2007) to the art of crafting "sticky" stories, ones that people cannot forget.

Examples convince. Fear a doubtful reviewer. Examples reassure that you are expert in your area and understand what you propose doing. Think of an application like a job interview. The more specific you are, the more convincing you are. During an interview, would you only say, "I'm good at research"? Or would you back that statement up with examples? Do the same in your proposal.

The eventual success of your application depends partly on how much reviewers believe you. They want you to guide them. They search for reassurance and are disquieted when they do not find it. So reach out your hand, take theirs, and show them the detailed world of your ideas. The examples you share are worth the space.

7.6 Eliminate Abbreviations

Consider this sentence, which is a modified version of an actual statement of objectives from a research grant.

The objective of this proposal is to evaluate how much the new USPSTF CPGs for prevention of CVD using ACC/AHA PCEs in patients with DM have been adopted among VHA providers.

The writer thought this was as clear as mountain spring water. To an outside reader, the sentence is mud. (To brush off some of that mud, here are what the abbreviations mean: USPSTF = United States Preventive Services Task Force, CPG = clinical practice guideline, CVD = cardiovascular disease, ACC = American College of Cardiology, AHA = American Heart Association, PCEs = pooled cohort equations [statistical tools], DM = diabetes mellitus, and VHA = Veterans Health Administration.) The writer saved room, but at what cost?

Yes, proposals often have strict page limits. Yes, you conserve space wherever possible. Yes, abbreviations (acronyms and initialisms) condense terms. And, as the example illustrates, abbreviations are risky.

Acronyms are abbreviations pronounced as words, such as SCUBA. Initialisms are abbreviations pronounced as letters, such as ATM. In either case, none of the combinations meant anything until they were created. Both are initially often discipline-specific. These abbreviations must be drummed, through endless repetition, into common usage. This takes time, even within a particular field. No matter how commonly used or catchy you think your abbreviations are, there are reviewers who do not know them or will not remember them. So you can cross your fingers. Or you can delete the abbreviations.

Even knowing this, most proposal writers consider their own abbreviations helpful. But no matter how stunning or inventive the letter combination might be, unknown abbreviations make reviewers stumble. Asking people who read your application as fast as possible, perhaps skimming parts, to memorize an abbreviation is like asking them to do you a big favor. Burning through multiple big favors rapidly diminishes a reviewer's goodwill.

Here are tips to help eliminate abbreviations in an application.

Set a rule. I suggest shooting for only three frequently used abbreviations per proposal. Write everything else out. Do *not* count those that you are *one hundred percent sure* everyone knows. If your country or the funding organization has an abbreviation for its name, for example, explain its meaning the first time, then employ it freely. Using only three abbreviations per application sounds difficult. You may assume your own abbreviations are necessary, important, and comprehensible when, at the same time, other people's frustrate you. The reviewers are your other people. Curb your use of abbreviations by setting a limit *before* you start writing.

Count the number of times you employ an abbreviation. Some proposals introduce an abbreviation and never use it again. Pick up your organization's publications or a previous proposal and count how many times abbreviations are used. Some may appear only two or three times. Remember the rule in the previous paragraph?

Search for how your abbreviations are spread out. Abbreviations cause strain if infrequently used. If you introduce a new abbreviation on the first page, most people will not recall what you mean when they see it again on the fifth page. Ask an outside reader to review what you believe is understandable. Then, listen to their honest answer and review the first rule again.

Save space in other ways. There are many techniques for tightening an application without resorting to abbreviations. Chapter 14 gives tips on how to edit and save space.

7.7 Use Short Sentences

I once polled a select group of top scientists for their thoughts on grant writing. The respondents for this unscientific sample were medical doctors and PhDs, each with millions of dollars in funding from an alphabet soup of organizations in the US and UK (Agency for Healthcare Research and Quality, The Commonwealth Fund, United Kingdom's National Institute for Health Research, US Department of Veterans Affairs, US National Institutes of Health, US National Science Foundation, and Patient-Centered Outcomes Research Institute, to name only a few). These individuals had careers in fields as diverse as astrophysics, implementation science, geriatrics, and psychophysiology. To investigate what promotes cognitive ease, I asked them several questions, including how to recognize poor and great prose in grant applications. One of the points all participants agreed on was sentence length.

When identifying the distinguishing characteristics of *poor* writing, the scientists wrote things such as the following: "Long sentences," "Long, garbled sentences," "Compound sentences," "Excessively long sentences," and "Sentence structure that's more than two lines."

When asked to identify central characteristics of *great* writing, they noted these features: "No convoluted sentences," "Succinct, specific sentences with few embedded clauses," "Using only as many words as needed," "Sentences are not too long," and "Short, clear sentences with SVO [subject, verb, object] organization."

Remember the coat hanger analogy from the 1–3-2/2–3-1 principle (Chap. 7, Sect. 7.1)? The reader who has the hanger (subject and verb) early on can easily organize the remainder of a sentence. Long introductory phrases and clauses pile clothes in readers' arms without giving them any way to arrange them. Cognitively, this is a burden. Too much of that, and a reader loses track of ideas or, worse, puts the material down.

Composing short sentences sounds easy. But long explanations allure, particularly when you delve into complex subject matter. Here is a five-step program to help you write short, concise sentences.

Step 1: Admit you have a problem. As a survey respondent noted, "Write in English everybody can understand." That means *everybody*. Not just you. Assess your level of addiction to lengthy phrasing. Drag out a recent document you wrote, a wordy email you sent, or any other substantial piece of writing you authored. Put a tick (or have AI put a tick) next to every long or convoluted sentence. Count the ticks.

Step 2: Make a commitment to practice regularly. Every day presents many opportunities to practice the craft of short sentences. One survey participant advised, "Pretend every word you write costs you a quarter." Implement that advice daily. The more you focus on precise, clear language in all your communication, the more you will employ it in your proposals.

Step 3: Learn from others. Colleges and universities realize that long sentences strain readers. They have websites to help. Search online for "how to write concise sentences" to discover practical tips. AI can dissect your text and suggest edits. Colleagues or books might serve as other sources of inspiration. Study examples you admire and mimic their style.

Step 4: Write for the right audience. A survey respondent recommended, "Write [proposals] for your high school science teacher. That's the right level." Notice what this means. You assume an intelligent reader who is familiar with the fundamentals of a field. But a science teacher is not a specialist. Imagine yourself at a high school reunion, explaining the essence of your proposal to this teacher. You will not dumb things down inaccurately but may simplify. You might use analogies, break complex ideas apart, or create a verbal diagram. That type of thinking will also help you write.

Step 5: Be your own harshest critic. This returns to Step 1. You will not try to improve if you think your long sentences are comprehensible. Leave attachment to your own writing style behind. Take the spontaneous responses of top scientists to heart. Learn how to edit your own work and proofread (see Chap. 14).

One survey question read as follows: "Imagine an intelligent, hard-working person comes to you with a expertly written document. Describe how you would recognize it as expertly written. What would you notice?" An answer: "It was clear, concise, and short." Practicing what they preached, that is all this person wrote.

7.8 Embrace your Reviewer

A critical first step in improving proposal writing involves embracing a reviewer as a living person, someone in front of you in a grocery store checkout line, with all the small and large struggles and successes of everyday life on their shoulders. A reviewer is an ordinary person with an important responsibility.

Exercise: Imagine Your Reviewer
Proposal writing is primarily a left-brain task. Pictures, on the other hand, are primarily processed in the brain's right side. So try creating a mental image of your reviewer. *Visualize* your answers to the following questions. Finish one before moving to the next. Be creative. Let your right brain participate.

1. *What does your reviewer do for a living?* What things in their environment reflect their job?
2. *Where do they perform the review?* What do you see? A quiet office? A kitchen table? An airport lounge?
3. *How did they prepare for reviewing the grant?* What do they have with them that reflects their preparation?
4. *Does your reviewer enjoy the task of reviewing grants?* How does their body language convey their emotional state? How do they hold their head, neck, back, arms, hands?
5. *What facial expression do they have while reading your grant?* What do their eyes, mouth, and forehead look like?
6. *What distracts the reviewer when reviewing your grant?* How do they limit those distractions? How do they react when intrusions break through?
7. *Where does your reviewer go when they need a break from grant reviewing?* What do they do there?
8. *If your reviewer had a pet, what would that be?*

How does the reviewer come to life in your answers? Does a representative trait or image stand out? How would you describe them to a friend?

Having an image of a real person in mind combats a difficulty that all grant writers struggle with: the blinder effect of external constraints. External constraints include limits on time, resources, and length (a proposal's maximum length is often limited by the funding organization). Separately and together, these pressures function as blinders and endanger success. They narrow a writer's focus to only the tasks ahead, making it difficult to see the larger picture of what happens after an application is submitted. This means that the greater the pressure, the less time a writer spends considering a reviewer's cognitive ease.

Think of a horse. Eons ago, horses were prey animals that required constant vigilance to avoid becoming a predator's meal. Over millennia, their head shape and eyes evolved to effectively scan their environment. Horses' brains constantly process enormous amounts of visual data, searching, in part, for predators. This still benefits horses in the wild. But for horses in task-oriented situations like running a race or pulling a carriage, all the data can be distracting, even dangerous.

Blinders help a horse focus on its task (the path ahead) and not see distractions that might unnecessarily scare it (other horses, humans, traffic). They limit a horse's field of vision, reducing the amount of data the horse needs to process, relaxing the horse and enabling it to concentrate.

Proposal writers need blinders from time to time, to limit distractions and improve focus. Experienced writers often create their own blinders. They block dedicated hours on their schedule, shut down email and the internet, avoid meetings, and sit behind a closed physical or virtual door. In such an environment, the quality of their thinking and writing increases.

But grant writers may also wear involuntary, detrimental blinders. Deliberately setting aside time to work on an application differs from *unintentionally* ignoring a reviewer's cognitive ease because time, resources, or text space is short. When, "I have to finish this proposal!" echoes ever louder, we tend to close ourselves off from other information, producing *invisible* blinders. The stronger the external pressures are, the larger these hidden blinders grow. We then default to the easiest course, which is ignoring the reviewer's experience.

Yet grant writers possess mindfulness, intelligence, and a capacity for both creativity and reason. They can combat the predictable pressures of external constraints with techniques and skills that promote focus without reducing clarity and breadth. Block time, eliminate distractions, and close a door. Remove your own stressors so you can create less stress for your reviewer.

References

Clark, R. P. (2006). *Writing Tools: 50 Essential Strategies for Every Writer*. Little, Brown and Company.

Heath, C., & Heath, D. (2007). *Made to Stick: Why Some Ideas Survive and Others Die*. Random House.

Kahneman, D. (2011). *Thinking, Fast and Slow*. Farrar, Straus, and Giroux.

Chapter 8
Building an Argument

Listening to young children tell stories requires patience. The stories meander, often following no perceptible structure or linear chronology. Background information is frequently missing. Digressions abound. The results can be amusing and sweet.

But adult brains search for orientation. We long for a logical flow. Proposals should provide that. Yet many writers skip the easiest step for building this: constructing an outline.

8.1 Outline Everything First

A basic grant outline consists only of sections, headings, and subheadings. You may be tempted to eschew this outline and simply begin writing sentences. But specifying your organizing terms *before* writing longer text enables faster editing. We all become attached to our words. The more words you write, the greater the likelihood you will find them difficult to change, reorganize, or delete. Yet careful editing is critical to successful proposal writing. A short outline of words or phrases is much easier to edit than sentences or paragraphs.

A list of sections, headings, and subheadings also forces you to condense your argument to its essentials. The outline covers what you want your reviewers to remember and how you will persuade them. In other words, it silhouettes the bones of an application and highlights its early flaws.

As covered in Chap. 7, Sect. 7.2, proposal writers often have difficulty identifying deficiencies that a reviewer may catch. An outline addresses this problem by revealing a proposal's infrastructure. The brevity of an outline enables you to assess content with relative detachment.

Building a strong outline involves four steps.

First, create a scaffold based on the funding organization's specifications. Read the request for applications or other solicitation documents to determine required

C. W. Hartmann, *Grant Writing Fundamentals Made Easy*,
https://doi.org/10.1007/978-3-032-35723-6_8

content and funding organization priorities. Also locate the review criteria, the standards by which reviewers will judge the proposal. Combine these to construct a draft of the proposal's sections. AI can help. Sections often follow a predictable order: background, supporting evidence, and prior studies; methods, analysis, and evaluation; dissemination, sustainment, and future work. But do not feel completely constrained by convention. Your primary audience is the reviewer. Organize your scaffold (or the one AI created for you) to make the reviewer's process easy by accentuating all requirements and review criteria.

Second, add details. The initial scaffold is generic, in that it could apply to any grant written for that funding organization's request. The next step involves adding details that apply to your specific ideas. Flesh out your argument, using descriptive words, not simply facts. Ask yourself the following questions and include their answers as you add headings and subheadings, section by section: How does this support my main argument? What should a reviewer believe after reading this? In what order do reviewers need to understand things?

Heading Examples

Headings and subheadings are descriptive steppingstones for a reviewer. They summarize the content that follows them, ideally highlighting the take home points, thereby forming a high-level logical path to follow. Embrace the use of full sentences, facts, and emotional punch in your headings. Strong headings and subheadings enable a reviewer to read only them and still get a clear idea of your main arguments. This benefits you because some reviewers may skim your proposal, reading only the headings, and because headings and subheadings come first, so reviewers are more likely to remember them. (See Chap. 7, Sect. 7.1 for more about the importance of placing important information first.)

Here are before and after versions of headings. What do you notice about how they engage you? Which ones prompt you to care about an issue? Are there some that make you want to read more?

Before: Effects of cancer screening with low-dose computed tomography.
After: Low-dose computed tomography reduces lung cancer mortality by 20%.
Before: Relationship of antimicrobial multidrug resistance to treatment.
After: Antimicrobial multidrug resistance complicates the treatment of many infectious diseases, with potentially life-threatening consequences.
Before: Older adults are an important population.
After: Adults over 75 represent one of largest, fastest growing, and most medically complex populations.

Tips for creating engaging headers include incorporating the subsequent text's punch line in the header, writing full sentences with active verbs, and including compelling details. Always ask yourself whether a reviewer can read only your headings and understand your main points.

Third, begin and end with your most important points. Follow the 1–3-2 principle from Chap. 7, Sect. 7.1. Use it overall and at the heading and subheading levels. Reviewers *will* skim. Put time into organizing for effect. Acknowledge that this is a strange goal—investing hours writing an application so reviewers can spend as little time as possible reading and understanding it. But this is the world in which proposal review takes place.

Fourth, edit. Outlines create an overview of your entire grant. Critically appraise that overview. Read it aloud. Share it with someone *not* familiar with it. Have AI dissect it. Does it make sense? Are the arguments convincing?

Outlining requires iterative editing. You draft an initial order, then reorder, add additional information, or delete. If a point lacks evidence, remove it and reconfigure the flow. When in doubt, subdivide points for clarity and include more evidence. Ensure that you meet all requirements of the funding organization. Also, ask an outside reader to assess whether you create a coherent trail to follow.

Move to the next stage by writing sentences and paragraphs anywhere in the outline. If you only have fifteen minutes, flesh out a subheading in the methods. If you have an hour, work on the significance or dissemination section. This process eases writer's block by breaking the grant into small pieces.

Avoid making the mistake of thinking outlines are juvenile or for people who do not have skill. Experienced grant writers use outlines. Why? Because reviewers need accurate and helpful sections, headings, and subheadings. When your reviewers skim your proposal—and they *will* skim it—a strong outline enables your argument to shine through and hands reviewers easy-to-find evidence they need to advocate for your work.

8.2 Determine Your Claim

Reviewers want a straightforward path to everything important, such as the current state of knowledge, prior activities of the team, and the potential effect of the project on something they value. They expect to be persuaded and satisfied. The fact-driven parts of their brains want answers.

If an application lacks logical reasoning, a reviewer may reread sentences or paragraphs or skip back and forth, causing cognitive strain. If the logic is disjointed enough, the reviewer may become annoyed. If their frustration grows, it can affect how carefully they read, increasing confusion and cognitive strain, resulting in more irritation. The best way to stop this cycle is to avoid what triggers it.

Every proposal makes a central claim about a subject, an assertion that hooks the reader and guides the subsequent text. There are several types of claims. One is a claim of fact. For example, "In the US, fewer children are illiterate now than twenty years ago." This claim can be shown to be true (data show there is less illiteracy) or untrue (data show there is more illiteracy). Other types of claims include a claim of value, such as, "Child illiteracy is unethical." This argument makes a value judgment. Another is a claim of policy, such as, "The US government should provide more funding to support early childhood education programs." This is a recommendation for action in a policy arena. In proposals, a claim of fact is most common.

Exercise: Discover Your Claim

Find a quiet space where you have access to a dictation or voice recording app.

Imagine yourself in a fancy Las Vegas hotel elevator on your way to a rooftop restaurant. An important person from your potential funding organization scoots in before the doors shut. You recognize them and introduce yourself. They perk up when they hear about your background and share that they have a discretionary pot of money for which you could apply. You have only 30 more seconds before the doors open again. Convince them that they should fund your claim. What is your elevator pitch?

Claims are neither true nor believable by default. A proposal's job is to assemble accurate evidence to convince. Most claims comprise multiple components.

Take, for example, a grant about planting trees. This may rest on three components if it makes the claim that planting ten trees per city block will benefit residents by (1) reducing noise pollution, (2) promoting safer driving habits, and (3) improving the environment. This example's underlying assumptions (things taken for granted) are that cities want to improve the living conditions for their inhabitants and that reducing noise pollution, promoting safer driving habits, and improving the environment are worthy goals. In other words, constructing a logical argument requires not only upholding claims but also explicitly stating and supporting underlying assumptions.

Once you clarify your claims and assumptions, write them down in a funnel order (from broad to specific) that makes sense for a naive reader. At the same time, collect evidence to reinforce them. Evidence can be statistics, data, prior studies, existing literature, a successful history, assertions of experts, specific examples, or relevant anecdotes. Do not insert claims or assumptions that do not have evidence. Once you have an ordered list, AI can assist with constructing multiple versions that you refine before choosing a final order that works best.

When describing evidence, be accurate. Sometimes, results from the literature or even your own prior studies are equivocal. Counterclaims may exist. If your subject lends itself to this type of controversy, your application should address it directly, describing the evidence and explaining the logic of your position. Assume your reviewers are familiar with this state of the science. Even if they are not, using words and phrases such as "suggests" or "points to" (instead of "shows" or "proves") indicates that you understand where your work is positioned. Underscore what your project adds and how that addition is important to a reviewer and the funding organization.

The bigger the point, or the more controversial or expansive it is, the more evidence you require for backing it up. Consider these two examples: "Urban trees *contribute to* the good health of a city's population" and "Urban trees *cause* the good health of a city's population." The former needs much less evidence than the latter. In the first statement, urban trees are only one of a range of contributors. In the second, they are the only contributor.

8.3 Create a Logical Flow

At a 30,000-foot level, a proposal's logic, and therefore its outline, most commonly follows the shape of a downward facing funnel. Broad claims and assumptions come first, along with their supporting evidence. As the narrative continues, claims and assumptions narrow in focus, as does their evidence. The funnel shape ends with the particulars of your approach. Other organizational styles exist. But breaking with the standard downward funnel (or its close cousin, the hourglass) requires experience and justification and should only be done if a classic funnel does not meet the proposal's needs.

Funneling from general to specific has several advantages.

A broad beginning entices a wider audience. Organizing from broad to specific hooks readers by acknowledging the extended implications of the work. Reviewers tend to come from diverse backgrounds and may not possess the insider awareness required to understand the minutiae of a proposal's aims. A more general start coaxes a reviewer to keep reading, particularly if it homes in on why they should care about the topic. How does this affect the world they know? What good or bad thing could happen if the application is funded or not funded? As the text progresses and narrows in scope, successive parts can dive into specifics necessary for understanding each deeper level.

The only caution for a broad beginning is to stay within the boundaries of what your project can achieve. Do not overpromise a relationship at the beginning of a proposal that you cannot justify at the end. For example, avoid leading with statistics related to reducing highway fatalities when your proposal is about investigating a chemical that *might*, ten or more years down the road, be used to study car tire traction under particular conditions. Remain within the scope of what is realistically related, something a reviewer can understand, believe, and use to justify your work in a review committee meeting.

A broad beginning can also encompass every aspect of a proposal's premise. Proposals often rest on multiple foundations. They might address more than one fundamental issue, require a specific set of methods, and/or depend on the collaboration of a particular team of individuals or organizations. A wider beginning can pull all these strands together.

When constructed logically, downward funnel organization leads a reader to believe the project is a reasonable solution to the issues at hand. When outlining the logical flow, think about the ultimate aims and work backward. What needs to precede the proposal's key aim(s)? What information does a reviewer require to believe the aim(s) will succeed? What arguments will persuade a reviewer? In what order? To answer these questions, think like an outsider to your topic. What would they dispute? Reviewers often wonder about the following.

1. Why should anyone care about this issue? This is the all-important "So what?" question.
2. What do we already know about it?

3. What do we not yet know? Where is an interesting area for investigation and discovery?
4. How do the key aim(s) of the proposal address what we do not know?
5. Why are the proposed methods the right ones?
6. Who is going to do the work? What has this team done before?
7. How will we know if the project worked?
8. How will this work be sustained, spread, or add to future work?

Answering these questions, in this approximate order, shapes the downward funnel. The answers are particularly helpful when crafting the section that provides background information, but the questions generally pertain throughout the entirety of a grant application.

If a proposal targeted at a local foundation argues for planting more trees along City Anywhere's streets, it may have the aim of planting ten trees per city block. In that case, the prior questions and answers might form a funnel like this.

1. Why should anyone care about this issue? So what?
   - The proposal could claim that trees along streets provide benefits, including reducing noise pollution, promoting safer driving habits, and improving the environment. (Let us call these points "A," "B," and "C," respectively).
     - Of course, you will include facts, data, and citations to back up these claims, as described in Sect. 8.2.
     - Consider including a brief story, anecdote, or quote if it is relevant and adds emotional impact.
2. What do we already know about the issue?
   - With three points to address, this part will be broken into at least three subsections, potentially more.
   - The answers will provide details and facts about A, B, and C, driving home their importance, particularly in relation to the aim of the proposal. For A it will describe evidence for how trees reduce noise pollution, etc.
     - These answers should also describe the current state of these issues relating to City Anywhere. How bad is noise pollution? What are the auto accident rates? What do we know about the city's environment?
   - In some cases, the answers to #1 and #2 may be combined. After introducing A, B, and C briefly, subsequent subheadings could address 1 and 2 for A in detail, then 1 and 2 for B, and 1 and 2 for C.
3. What do we not yet know? Where is an interesting area for investigation and discovery?
   - The proposal could explain that we do not know what will happen in City Anywhere if we plant trees and how and why this is a beneficial area for investigation.

4. How do the key aim(s) of the proposal address what we do not know?
    - At this stage of the funnel, a reviewer understands A, B, and C, the relevant evidence, and the need for investigation. So this answer could be, for example, that the evidence presented in #2 shows that similar cities have planted ten trees per block and demonstrated improvement in areas A, B, and C, so this project has a firm foundation for moving ahead with tree planting in City Anywhere and will monitor outcomes over time to see if the city experiences the same benefits.
5. Why are the proposed methods the right ones?
    - The answer should show that the project considers both what is known and what could go wrong.
    - Perhaps the team has contacted similar cities and compiled a list of what worked and what did not and why. It could describe methods that build off this knowledge and include contingency plans for potential known obstacles.
    - The thrust of the answer provides evidence for the choices made.
6. Who is going to do the work? What has this team done before?
    - This answer, for example, may describe a special collaboration of organizations that have had historical success in working together on city projects.
    - Both the team and the prior projects can be described in further sections, as dictated by the requirements for a particular application.
7. How will we know this project worked?
    - This question is about evaluation. The answer covers plans for that.
    - In this case, it could involve a description of data the city already collects that will determine whether there is improvement in A, B, and C.
8. How will this work be sustained, spread, or add to future work?
    - The answer could explain that the project rests on reliable, existing funding sources that will cover expenses associated with tree planting, such as watering, pruning, and replacing. The results of the monitoring, if positive, could provide additional evidence to help other cities implement similar programs.

8.4 Scrutinize for Gaps in Logic

Even when creating detailed funnels, logical fallacies and gaps in logic may be difficult for a writer to see. Yet these often spring out to a reviewer who is on the hunt for counterexamples and flaws.

8.4.1 Logical Fallacies

As a writer, it helps to keep several common logical fallacies in mind to sensitize yourself to their potential presence. The examples given are simple. Each of these fallacies can also appear in complex contexts and be more difficult to spot.

Circular reasoning involves using your own claim as evidence to support it. "Child illiteracy affects children's social interactions in school because when children cannot read, it affects how they interact with others." This statement makes the same claim twice, without evidence. A stronger one would be, "One reason child illiteracy affects children's social interactions in school has to do with the many written social cues in a school environment. Research shows that children who fail to perceive these cues modify their interactions to cope with and/or hide their confusion."

Generalizing has two parallel types. Hasty generalization involves jumping to a conclusion despite limited or inadequate factual support. "A prior study with ten children showed an accelerated reading program improved literacy. All schools should therefore use this program." A sweeping generalization is similar and assumes that something that works in a particular context will work everywhere. "A prior study in a private school showed that an accelerated reading program improved literacy. We are therefore going to use this same program in all public schools in our district."

Not following is when a claim is not supported by the evidence presented. "Studies show children's social interactions improve when they learn to read. Therefore, all schools in our district should increase teacher pay."

Incorrect chronological assumption involves assuming that because something happened *after* something else, the two are linked by cause and effect. "We implemented a pilot reading program in the school for three weeks in September. The following January, most students' reading scores had improved."

Black and white fallacy is when you set up a claim as though there are only two options (black and white) when there are, actually, many possibilities. "Child illiteracy rates drive adult poverty rates."

Some problems with logic do not involve fallacies. Logic problems may present as jumps, omissions, or disorganization. These can be harder to see, particularly for subject matter experts, who may fill in gaps in their heads. To further understand what problems with logic can look like, it may help to examine an example from an actual proposal's background-providing section. This application focused on improving blood pressure care for Black individuals by tailoring interventions to ethnic backgrounds (Black people from Caribbean countries, Africa, Guyana, etc.). The initial flow contains several logic jumps. The revision improves the flow. I also present the revision as a table, with annotations that indicate why each point is logically necessary. As with most aspects of grant writing, there is not one correct answer. What might you might do similarly or differently and why?

8.4.1.1 Initial Flow

1. High blood pressure in the US population is prevalent; it is disproportionately prevalent among Black individuals.
2. Digital health technology (remote patient monitoring) has the potential to improve high blood pressure self-management.
3. There is low uptake of remote patient monitoring among Black individuals compared with other groups.
4. Social determinants of health are used as explanations for these disparities.
5. Current research efforts that look at social determinants of health are not sufficient to explain low uptake.
6. Additional factors, such as ethnic background among Black individuals, might help explain disparities.

STOP. Read the flow again and say aloud where you see jumps in logic. How would you edit this outline? Why would you make each change?

After you have finished, read the revision, noting how it is similar to or different from your edits.

8.4.1.2 Revised Outline

1. High blood pressure in the US population is prevalent; it is disproportionately prevalent among Black individuals.
2. Black individuals have worse outcomes related to high blood pressure.
3. Self-management is a critical component for improving outcomes.
4. Digital health technology (remote patient monitoring) has the potential to improve high blood pressure self-management and outcomes.
5. There is low uptake of remote patient monitoring among Black individuals.
6. Social determinants of health are used as explanations for low uptake of remote patient monitoring.
7. Current research efforts looking at social determinants of health are not sufficient to explain the low uptake of remote patient monitoring.
8. Healthcare interventions similar to remote patient monitoring that acknowledged ethnic heterogeneity among Black individuals had improved uptake.
9. Acknowledging ethnic heterogeneity is thus likely to improve uptake of remote patient monitoring.
10. We therefore need to investigate how best to incorporate ethnic heterogeneity in remote patient monitoring interventions for Black individuals so we can evaluate whether this promising avenue works to improve uptake and self-management and thereby improves outcomes.

Table 8.1 shows the revision with annotations about the rationale for each point.

Cultivating the ability to diagnose logical fallacies and other problems with logic represents one of the most demanding tasks for a proposal writer. It requires a

Table 8.1 Annotated revision

Point	Rationale
1. **High blood pressure** in the US population is prevalent; it is disproportionately prevalent among **black individuals.**	Sets up the **disease area** and the **population.**
2. Black individuals have **worse outcomes** related to high blood pressure.	Sets up the **pressing issue**. Because of this, for the first sentence of the proposal, it might help to combine outline points 1 and 2, or have 1 immediately precede 2, so the reader at once understands the disease, population, and issue.
3. **Self-management** is a critical component for improving outcomes.	**Sets up self-management as a critical, necessary component** to address the issue. This is necessary because remote patient monitoring does not improve the outcome directly but by improving self-management. Self-management is therefore the critical link between the outcome that drives reviewer interest and the intervention (remote patient monitoring) that drives the proposal.
4. Digital health technology (**remote patient monitoring**) has been shown to improve high blood pressure self-management and outcomes.	Working through the sentence, remote patient monitoring is "B," self-management is "C," and outcomes is "D." (do not worry. "A" appears below.) this sets up that B leads to C and D (B➔C➔D).
5. There is **low uptake** of remote patient monitoring among black individuals.	**Critical issue for investigation**
6. **Social determinants of health are used** as explanations for low uptake of remote patient monitoring.	How people have traditionally thought about this issue.
7. Current research efforts looking at s**ocial determinants of health are not sufficient** to explain the low uptake of remote patient monitoring.	But thinking up to now **does not actually explain the critical issue.**
8. Healthcare interventions similar to remote patient monitoring that acknowledged **ethnic heterogeneity** among black individuals had improved uptake.	But we probably *do* know how to address this issue if we look at similar healthcare interventions that acknowledged ethnic heterogeneity and have had success (this is "A"). This sets up that A➔B➔C➔D.
9. **Acknowledging ethnic heterogeneity is thus likely to improve uptake** of remote patient monitoring.	**Acknowledging ethnic heterogeneity is a likely answer to addressing the critical issue.**
10. We **therefore need to investigate how best to acknowledge ethnic heterogeneity in remote patient monitoring interventions for black individuals** so we can evaluate whether this promising avenue works to improve uptake and self-management and thereby improves outcomes.	This study should be done. Everything points to the need to investigate (1) how best to acknowledge ethnic heterogeneity and then (2) pilot test a new way to address it. We think it is highly likely to succeed, based on the logic of A➔B➔C➔D.

distanced stance and an ability to enter the mind of a reader who lacks any familiarity with the details of the application. Few people do this consistently, which is why enlisting the help of outside readers (see Chap. 4, Sect. 4.4) or AI at this stage is critical.

8.5 Consider Using a Logic Model

A logic model is a diagram of a project's resources, activities, and results. It can provide reviewers and funders with a clear map for understanding the relationship between what you plan to do and what will result. It often comprises inputs, activities, outputs, and outcomes, with these subdivided as appropriate. It may also include risks and mitigation strategies. Many examples exist online. Find what works for you and your project. As with other graphics (see Chap. 11, Sect. 11.7), this visual depiction, when done well, can clarify relationships and provide a quick understanding that is not possible using only text. A logic model can be an easy-to-find, valuable asset for reviewers to appreciate and defend your work.

8.6 Understand your Audience

Just as business marketers pitch a product according to how much potential customers know about it, proposals benefit from understanding a reviewer's awareness of the issues an application focuses on. I adapted Mike Kim's levels of consumer awareness from his book *You are the Brand* (2021) to create four levels of grant reviewer awareness.

8.6.1 Level 1

At this level, a reviewer does not realize there is a problem or is not familiar with the issue. The first sentences should therefore raise a reviewer's awareness. In an example from earlier, not everyone understands that trees benefit urban environments. If you think your reviewers will be unfamiliar with this broader context, educate and convince them. Define the problem to arouse a reviewer's curiosity. For example, "In just one year, a single mature tree absorbs over forty-eight pounds of carbon dioxide from the air, replacing it with oxygen that can offset air pollution sources in cities." This statement focuses on one benefit of trees and the possibilities of planting trees in cities. Subsequent sentences can home in on other benefits.

8.6.2 Level 2

At Level 2, reviewer realizes there is a problem but does not know of a solution. In this case, the first sentences emphasize that your proposal presents a solution to the known problem or issue. In the tree example, an approach could be the following: "Urban trees reduce noise pollution, promote safer driving habits, and improve the environment, making trees an effective, low-cost solution to address some of modern cities' most intractable issues." Again, you must define the solutions to enable reviewers to follow your next steps.

8.6.3 Level 3

A Level 3 reviewer understands solutions exist but does not know of your solution or does not recognize which solution to choose. The initial sentences for this level can highlight the unique benefits of your solution or method. For example, "Cities all over the world implement countless interventions for problems associated with urban living. But no intervention offers more benefits at relatively low cost than the simple one of planting trees."

8.6.4 Level 4

At this highest level, a reviewer knows of your solution and likes it. The beginning sentences therefore focus on what you, and only you, can deliver. "Efficient and effective planting and maintenance of urban trees requires a multidisciplinary, community-involved approach, which is what our team brings to this project."

As is clear in these examples, how you describe information depends on what you believe reviewers' level of awareness is. No one has a crystal ball to show who reviewers are and what they know. But writers can make educated guesses based on the funding organization's priorities and the general state of knowledge about a topic. Reviewers at Level 1, for example, need sufficient background to appreciate the relevance of an issue. For them, a proposal written only to Level 4 will be confusing.

When in doubt about how much your reviewers might know, pitching to Level 1 awareness is a safe bet. No reviewer ever complained, "This proposal was too easy to understand."

Reference

Kim, M. (2021). *You Are the Brand*. Morgan James.

Chapter 9
The Proposal's Hook

I uncovered the connection between screenwriting and grant writing relatively late in my career. It began when I stumbled on the screenwriter's bible, the book *Story: Substance, Structure, Style, and the Principles of Screenwriting*, by Robert McKee (1997). I devoured its principles for creating drama. Later, in McKee's virtual seminars, I learned what underpins a riveting narrative.

A great film hooks an audience through an early event that raises an exciting question. The search for answers drives the characters and viewers through the rest of the story. The horror film *Get Out* grips crowds with its first scene: the backdrop of racial injustice frames the violence of a stranger attacking and abducting a Black man walking through a White neighborhood. In the animated film *Frozen*, Elsa accidentally misuses her power to turn matter into ice, injuring her sister and setting off an eternal winter. Whether Elsa will bring her power under control drives the subsequent story.

In the cinematic world, this crucial early inflection point is called the inciting incident. It represents the moment at which the plot becomes compelling because something important in the lives of the central figures is out of kilter. The audience cannot look away until they learn whether or how balance will be restored. Screenwriters understand the importance of the inciting incident and the story arc it sets into motion.

Grant writers benefit from employing the same tactic, which in the grant writing world is called a "hook."

Reviewers are to grants what viewers are to films. A strong hook in a proposal, just like an inciting incident in a film, draws people in. It must immediately address a reviewer's questions, "So what? Why should I care?" To do this, it must meet

---

Parts of this chapter are used with permission of Springer Nature BV, from How screenwriting can help your grant writing, Christine W. Hartmann, *Nature*. 2023 Jun 7; permission conveyed through Copyright Clearance Center, Inc.

C. W. Hartmann, *Grant Writing Fundamentals Made Easy*,
https://doi.org/10.1007/978-3-032-35723-6_9

two conditions related to the subject of the application. It must convey a sense of emotional urgency and open a question in the reviewer's mind (Hartmann, 2023).

Grant writers create emotional urgency by employing contrast, concretizing consequences, and showing the work's importance to reviewers' and funding organizations' worlds. They juxtapose effects of conducting versus not conducting the work. What will be better in the world if this project succeeds? What harms will it mitigate? What suffers if this work is not performed? Good hooks relate statistics to real-world issues. Numbers help. But numbers do not motivate unless they are tied to something concrete and meaningful.

When a reviewer reads something interesting that they do not know the answer to, a question opens in their mind. J.K. Rowling drove seven Harry Potter books based on readers wanting to know the answer to an idea conjured in the first chapter of the first book: When Voldemort meets Harry face-to-face, who will survive? In a grant, a well-written hook does not need to propel seven books. But the goal *is* to engage a reviewer enough to have them keep reading with interest.

9.1 Hooks for any Discipline

A successful proposal focuses on immediate or possible repercussions of a project, connecting these to facts or scenarios that energize a reviewer's feelings and help the reviewer connect the work to what the funding organization wants to see. But what if your research takes place in a lab or feels in other ways removed from everyday life? Maybe you specialize in inorganic chemistry or quantum physics. How do you connect to feelings when your project is distanced from an immediate emotional outcome? Does attempting to generate a sense of emotional urgency even make sense?

Many scientific disciplines avoid any discussion of feelings, particularly in grant applications. This distanced stance may be what researchers are taught. But a different perspective is possible and even desirable. Reviewers are human. They all have emotions and understand connections to larger pictures. Here are techniques for building emotional urgency in disciplines that—at first glance—have weaker associations with the world of feelings.

Connect to bigger-picture issues that are emotional or urgent. Sometimes research is foundational to answering broader questions. The subject itself may seem devoid of emotional topics. But a few steps down the road, the work might be used to improve important outcomes, policies, or regulations. Connect those dots. Underscore the significance of what you propose by showing how it helps discover something or moves a field toward a meaningful consequence or product. What potential transferability can you showcase? Can you demonstrate how results and the intellectual merit of the work advance issues that matter to reviewers and the funding organization? Avoid overselling or stretching beyond what is reasonable given the scope of the project. But draw reasonable and justified comparisons that may not be immediately apparent to a reviewer.

Identify what excites you about your work. What gets you into the office or lab in the morning? Why are you motivated to do your research? Determine those elements. Write them down as though you were explaining this at a party to a friend. Then, convey your own genuine excitement and interest in your grant.

Create an analogy that links your work to something reviewers understand. Ask your favorite AI software program, "What are some analogies for the importance of conducting research on [insert your line of scientific inquiry]?" The answers will likely be too broad for a hook. Continue the chat, asking AI to refine its answers to better match your specific field of research and/or to add more emotional punch. The results will likely provide a good starting point for crafting a compelling hook.

Tie your research to a scientific question that needs to be answered. Once you have done this, make the need compelling by explaining why answering this question is important. Why does it matter? Why is now the right time? What will move forward? Underscore the crucial/foundational/pivotal role your work plays in the journey.

Are there any precedents where your type of basic research served as the foundation for eventual other work that made an impact? Can you highlight a historical case, showing that projects such as yours could support meaningful future advancements?

If your work has many possibilities, create excitement about the unknowns. Opening a question in the mind of a reviewer and answering it over the course of an application is a successful technique for driving interest. For example, if in the future, your project could branch into three possible work streams, present this as positive. Explain how this occurs, why each of these streams is important, and how your project will determine the best future course. Keep in mind that a question is often implicit rather than explicit. A hook presents a scenario, and the reader wonders whether something great can be achieved or how a negative situation can be resolved.

If your work is an incremental but necessary step toward something else, why is now the right time to do it? Explain the gains of moving quickly. What does delaying risk? Create urgency.

A good hook evolves over time. You are not aiming for perfect. You are aiming for better than the previous version. Be precise and engaging. Choose wording to interest readers. Do not overstate or exaggerate your case. Create multiple versions. Ask someone outside your field to share their impressions of your ideas. Run the ideas through AI, asking AI to serve as a reviewer. Iteratively refine and evaluate the results.

Here are fictional first sentences (hooks) for a proposal's summary, with before and after versions, presented in alphabetical order by discipline. See if you can tell which technique applies to each "after" version.

Astrophysics A proposal about Moon dust.
Before: The electric field near the surface of the Moon, along with gravity, levitates dust.
After: Dust levitating above the Moon's surface poses risks to mechanical equipment.
Atomic Physics A proposal about the behavior of the gases of neutral atoms.

Before: This study develops theories that can guide future experimental detection of how gases of neutral atoms exhibit unusual behaviors under certain conditions.
After: The development of theories to explain how gases of neutral atoms exhibit unusual behaviors represents a fundamental step for supporting future developments in areas as diverse as navigation and information processing.
Biology A proposal about investigating biofilm infections.
Before: We do not understand the physical properties of biofilm infections.
After: To identify key targets for better medical treatment, we need to understand the physical properties of biofilm infections, which account for up to 80% of all human bacterial infections.
Education A proposal to fund the development of a semester-long course on intervening to prevent war.
Before: War seems an inevitable part of human culture, as even early artifacts record the existence of fighting among peoples.
After: Teaching about how to prevent wars without examining the cultural forces that support, shape, and repeat them is like training auto mechanics to repair engines without explaining how cars operate.
Health Sciences A proposal investigating the implementation of a new diabetes self-management app.
Before: This study will investigate the effectiveness of a novel diabetes self-management app.
After: Diabetes motivates our team, not only because it is one of the most devastating and disabling diseases, affecting over 830 million people globally, but also because it is highly amenable to self-management, an area where we can leverage considerable prior research, team expertise, and collaborations to make a difference.
Mechanical Engineering A proposal for developing better artificial cartilage for use in joint replacement surgeries.
Before: The intricate tissue of healthy cartilage helps lubricate and ease movement in joints.
After: Five percent of joint replacement surgeries fail within ten years, many due to wear and tear of the artificial cartilage.
Public Health A proposal about investigating how to prevent postpartum hypertension (high blood pressure).
Before: Many women suffer from postpartum hypertension.
After: The common condition of postpartum hypertension significantly increases a woman's risk of developing cardiovascular disease and depression, having a stroke, and dying.
Social Work A proposal about children with hearing impairment who are in foster care.
Before: Adjustment to foster care placement differs for children with normal hearing and those with hearing impairment.
After: Children in foster care with hearing impairment, when compared with those with normal hearing, are exponentially more likely to have worse placement outcomes.

Sociology A proposal to study, over time, students interested in machine learning. Before: We have no longitudinal data about students in two- and four-year degree programs who express an early interest in studying machine learning.
After: Today's world revolves around machine learning, necessitating an increasingly sophisticated workforce, yet we know nothing about why students who express initial interest in pursuing such a degree continue in or leave the field.

Experiment with which techniques align best with your work and application. Emotional urgency combines endlessly with engaging questions. A strong hook contains one or a few sentences that combine both. These involve a reviewer in your issue from the start and are possible to create for any discipline.

9.2 A Hook's Content

How do you build a short hook? There are two parts to the process: understanding your content and understanding your audience.

Exercise: Creating Content for a Hook
To each of the questions below, write or say aloud a one-sentence answer about your proposal.

1. What will change—in science, for a specific population, for your city, etc.—if your project is funded? (Be realistic; this must be credible change achievable during the funding period.) At a microbe/human/societal/etc. level, how will the world be a better place or what harms will be avoided if your claim comes true? (See Chap. 8, Sect. 8.2 for more about claims in proposal writing.) What answers the "So what? Why should I care?" questions?
2. How will we know the world is better? What statistics, people, programs, states of being, etc. will document added benefit or avoided harm?
3. Why do we not already know how to overcome the issues your proposal addresses? Why has this not been done before? What has stood in the way of progress, and how does your project address this?
4. Why is now the right time to do this work?
5. How does this work align with the funding organization's priorities?

Forcing yourself to answer each question in one sentence each creates five powerful statements. These form the underpinnings of your hook.

Imagine a proposal from a small nonprofit agency asking for funds from a state-based tourism board to help a beachside community reduce pollution along its shoreline. Here are example answers to the questions.

1. What will change? Studies show that cleaning up and preventing pollution improves beachgoers' experiences, reduces unnecessary seabird and sea creature injuries and deaths, and increases a community's tourist appeal.

2. How will we know the world is better? Communities that have implemented measures such as those proposed have experienced a 30% rise in beachgoer satisfaction scores, a 15% decrease in seabird and sea creature injuries, and a 20% increase in tourist spending.
3. Why do we not already know how to overcome these issues? Prior efforts have involved only limited areas of beachfront and have focused either on prevention or cleanup, while this proposal implements a large-scale approach targeting simultaneous prevention and cleanup, which was shown to be successful in similar communities.
4. Why is now the right time? This community is receiving increasing social media attention, which has the potential to boost tourism, but only if the beachfront is clean.
5. How does this work align with the funding organization's priorities? This project targets tourism and tourist satisfaction as key outcomes.

Combining these answers creates a strong draft first paragraph. But read on, because the order in which things are written can vary widely. And you can often incorporate the essence of multiple answers in one sentence.

9.3 A Hook's Audience

A reviewer's level of awareness (see Chap. 8, Sect. 8.6) guides the construction of a hook. If your issue is complex, understudied, or affects only a small but important group, you might assume your reviewers fall at Level 1 (not knowing there is a problem). If the underlying problem is well known but you are taking an unusual approach, you may assume your reviewers fall at Level 2 (knowing there is a problem but not knowing about solutions). If your problem is common knowledge and potential solutions are frequently in the news, you may assume your reviewers fall into Level 3 (knowing about solutions but not sure which is best). If you have already received money from this organization and are asking for an extension or additional funding, you may assume your reviewers fall at Level 4 (knowing and liking the solution you propose). Of course, as indicated elsewhere, reviewers within one review committee may fall into multiple groups. As also noted, writing to Level 1 is often a safe route.

For the shoreline pollution proposal above, where do you think reviewers from the state-based tourism board would fall? What if the proposal went instead to an automobile manufacturer's foundation that is interested in funding local projects across the nation? What would you change about the answers? What would you cut or add?

9.4 Drafting a Hook

To draft a hook, you can combine content and audience, engage emotions, and open a question. Returning to the shoreline pollution example, keep in mind the four content questions and the four levels of awareness. If the proposal were submitted to a state-based tourism board, you might assume reviewers fall into Level 3 of awareness. In that case, your hook may center on how this project will surmount the existing obstacles, since reviewers know of solutions but not why yours is best. You could still incorporate answers to other relevant content questions. But the first question to raise (and answer) is about how your project is the right one to overcome the outstanding issues. You could write, "Communities similar to ours have meaningfully improved the beachgoer experience, decreased wildlife injuries and death, and boosted tourism by employing the novel approach of simultaneously tackling both prevention and cleanup of shoreline pollution." The emotional effect is embedded in the three ways other communities have succeeded. The implicit question it opens is whether comparable results can be achieved. To boost the funding organization's priorities to the top, you could change this to, "Communities similar to ours have meaningfully boosted tourism and improved tourist experiences by employing the novel approach we propose here: that of simultaneously tackling both prevention and cleanup of shoreline pollution."

Using the same example, if the proposal went to a national automobile manufacturer's foundation, you would likely assume reviewers fall at Level 1 of awareness, not knowing a problem exists. In that case, you may want to focus predominantly on what will change. Again, incorporating answers to the other content questions will help flesh out your message. But the hook could first raise and answer the question of why change is important, since reviewers are likely not to know that. You might write, "Shoreline pollution takes a significant human, animal, and economic toll on our community." Or you might prefer an even shorter version, such as, "Shoreline pollution contributes to community decline." The emotional content comes from wondering what could be done to fix this.

Note that neither of the sample hooks integrates the answer to "why now." But they could. If you think timing is of the essence, include that. Here is one with "why now" incorporated: "Our popular social media profiles give increasing exposure to all aspects of our community, including the significant human, animal, and economic toll of our community's shoreline pollution." This version, however, hits the funding organization's priorities less directly. If you wanted to maintain the shorter hook (and shorter hooks are often desirable, as they promote cognitive ease), you could include the urgency piece in the next sentence. You could also include facts or statistics in any of these examples to bolster your case and make it more memorable. The options are endless.

There is no single best hook. Many writers revise and refine it over time. Be creative. Write several, because a proposal often requires hooks in various sections. Ask colleagues, friends, and AI to pretend they are the kind of reviewer you anticipate having. Which do they like best and why?

9.5 Where to Put a Hook and What Follows

Grant writing is like fishing, where the proposal writer sits in a boat holding a rod and line and the reviewer is a fish. The hook is the enticing bait at the end of the strand. Like bait, the hook must be visible. This means it should come at the beginning of a section. But which section? And what should follow to reel a reviewer in?

Obvious places for hooks include any high-level summary or overview. Depending on the funding organization, these sections may be an executive summary, a specific aims page, an overview, an abstract, a summary, or a statement of goals or objectives (see Chap. 10, Sect. 10.2 and Chap. 11, Sect. 11.2 for more on these parts of a proposal). These pieces always benefit from having a hook as the first sentence or sentences. A hook can also help define a letter of inquiry, letter of intent, or cover letter. Other, less apparent locations include the statement of need, the purpose of the request, and the impact, significance, and relevance sections.

Where you employ a hook depends mostly on how willing you are to break with convention. Traditional grant writing advice steers writers toward dry, less engaging openings for sections, ones that avoid touching reviewers' emotions or desire for knowledge. But compelling sections grab readers from the first sentences. A convincing grant benefits from multiple versions of a hook, each matching the intent of the section it begins.

Of course, to catch a fish, no one throws bait in the ocean without a line. A hook by itself without adequate support interests a reader only for a moment. Appropriate reinforcing sentences should follow.

Two elements define what constitutes appropriate follow-up: the hook's content and the content of the main aim(s). The hook is bait, but the goal of the application is to land a convinced reviewer in your boat. As illustrated in Chap. 8, Sect. 8.3, the sentences, paragraphs, and sections after the hook achieve that goal by creating a logical train of thought (the fishing line) that the reviewer follows from one point to the next, usually in the shape of a downward funnel.

In the above example, a proposal asks a state tourism board for funding to reduce shoreline pollution for a beachside community. The local organization wants to implement a two-pronged approach that has worked in similar communities. A fictional executive summary limited to two paragraphs could therefore begin with the following short hook.

"Shoreline pollution reduces tourism and negatively affects tourist experience and spending."

Pretend you must write the first paragraph of this executive summary, in which the second paragraph covers methods and other subjects. In the first paragraph, what will lead the reader from bait (hook) to boat (convinced)?

Imagine your initial outline looks like this.

1. Hook.
2. Introduce the successful strategy similar communities used: a two-pronged approach.
3. Give statistics on the positive effects of this two-pronged approach.

4. Cite statistics on how beachgoer experience is affected by shoreline pollution.
5. Describe similar statistics for wildlife and tourism.
6. End by saying we will use the two-pronged approach.

Does this outline use an inverted funnel approach? Do you see any gaps in logic? What would you change or add to have it comply more with what a reviewer needs to see? Take a moment to revise it, writing down or saying aloud your own version.

Now examine the second example, which creates a broad-to-narrow funnel and addresses logic gaps.

1. Hook.
2. Define shoreline pollution.
3. Explain why beachgoer experience is important to this community's tourism and how it is affected by shoreline pollution.
4. Explain how wildlife death affects this community's tourism.
5. Emphasize other effects of pollution on tourism.
6. Say what we have tried and why it has not worked.
7. Introduce a successful strategy similar communities used: a two-pronged approach.
8. Give statistics on the positive effect of this two-pronged approach.
9. Detail what is necessary for implementing this approach.
10. Document how we have methods, personnel, and expertise to do the same thing.
11. Say we propose to do this.

With approximately one sentence for each point, this revised paragraph would be about eleven sentences. What do you think? How is this revision similar to or different from your own? Does this paragraph move a reviewer from bait to boat? What would you change?

9.6 Starting with a Question

How do sea urchins reproduce? Why is a washing machine so heavy? Where do ocean waters get their salt? Do these questions grab you?

If they do, it is because you do not know the answer and are intrigued. Mysteries capture our attention, as Chip and Dan Heath describe in their book *Made to Stick: Why Some Ideas Survive and Others Die* (2007). When we recognize an interesting gap in our knowledge, we feel curious to know more. Critical to this "gap theory" of curiosity is that a gap needs to be opened before it can be closed. Imagine writing a proposal to fund research on sea urchin reproduction. Which of these sentences do you like better?.

A. Sea urchins rarely move and may not be near each other—so how do they reproduce?
B. Sea urchins reproduce by releasing sperm and eggs into the ocean around them.

Sentence A evokes curiosity and hooks a reviewer's attention. Sentence B erases curiosity. In the case of Sentence A, the proposal will provide the answer.

You can employ this technique across many different subject areas. Here are some example questions to spark a reviewer's curiosity along with the planned work that would provide a solution.

- *Why are children in our community not using public transportation to get to school?* An application proposes a project to improve lighting at bus stops.
- *What would you do if your mother were diagnosed with early-onset Alzheimer's disease?* The proposal investigates the success of a virtual group therapy intervention for children of people living with early-onset Alzheimer's disease.

Sometimes, however, a subject area is so specialized that writers must assume reviewers lack the background information to recognize an important gap even when it is presented. I review proposals on many different subjects related to healthcare organizations. But I know relatively little about human physiology. If I were to read a grant that began with the sentence, "What if we could develop a new technology for patients with glaucoma that could accurately image individual retinal ganglion cells?" the question would not hook me because I do not understand why accurate imaging of individual ganglion cells is needed. I cannot appreciate the gap.

In cases where reviewers might not recognize a gap, an applicant should provide context for the gap first. In the above example, this would involve helping reviewers understand why imaging individual retinal ganglion cells is critical. Here is a revision, where context precedes the gap. "In the eyes of glaucoma patients, retinal ganglion cells and their nerve fibers—which carry light signals to the brain—undergo progressive deterioration, leading to eventual vision loss. But not all cells deteriorate at the same timepoint. Early in the disease, some cells are completely normal and others are deteriorating but still functioning. Yet current imaging technologies cannot capture deterioration at the individual cell level. At-risk patients (those with some deteriorating cells) look the same as patients where all cells are normal. This prevents timely intervention with existing treatments to support deteriorating cells. What if we could develop an innovative technology to accurately image *individual* retinal ganglion cells, identifying cell-level deterioration and enabling us to start patients earlier on treatments to save vision?"

How do you react to this revision? In cases such as this, when reviewers need a longer setup (more information) to care about a gap, a proposal can employ a variant of the 1–3-2 principle, the 2–3-1 order. (See Chap. 7, Sect. 7.1 for more on this principle.) Lead with important background information and end with the question that hooks.

At first, including a question might feel uncomfortable. But I have seen many successful proposals employ this method. You may arouse more interest and curiosity with a question than a statement. Think of your own subject area. What intriguing questions could open gaps? Do these need an introduction or can they stand alone? Test ideas on colleagues and friends. Find the most exciting one and try it in your next proposal.

9.7 Fundamental Principles for Strong Hooks

Spending time crafting a hook pays off. Walking the line between too narrow and too broad, too grand and too boring, requires skill and experience. Four principles can assist you.

Shorter is generally better. Struggling through a long sentence with many clauses and tangents increases a reader's cognitive strain and lessens the likelihood that the hook will do what you want: turn the reader into a believer. If you need proof, look at the two sentences preceding this one, the one in italics and the next one. Think about their relative effects. The first is crisp and to the point. The second, while informative, takes longer to digest and packs less punch. In a sea of longer sentences, a short one carries weight. The converse, however, can also be true. Sometimes a longer sentence feels necessary. Shortening the sentences that precede or follow it gives it gravitas and makes it easier to absorb in context.

Focus on only the most important ideas. Pare down a hook until it highlights only the main points. Check for the use of introductory phrases or clauses and ideas linked with "and." You have an entire application to address nuances and secondary issues. Think of a hook as a command to your reviewer: "Believe this." Clarity and focus sharpen that command.

Never lead with a negative (like this). A negative statement includes "not," "never," or other negative words. (The revision of the italicized sentence here is, "Always lead with a positive.") Negative constructions mean a reader must digest the negative scenario to understand the positive. Anywhere in an application, negative construction can cause confusion and cognitive strain. Negative construction in a hook can lead to paradoxical results and make points more difficult to remember.

Test your hook. On a small scale, you might use the marketing technique of "A-B testing" by crafting at least two hooks (version A and version B) and evaluating them on a varied readership. Ask the readers to choose the most persuasive one. Be prepared to be surprised by their answers and willing to go with their choice if there is an overwhelming favorite.

9.8 Hook Revision Example

Below are three successive versions of a one-paragraph summary of the background-providing section of an application. In each, the hook is the first sentence (bolded). The remaining sentences hit other important points (see Sect. 9.2). As you read, speak aloud your answers to the following questions.

- Does the hook engage emotions and open a question?
- What hook and cognitive ease principles do the paragraphs embrace?
- When does a paragraph ignore a principle about hooks?
- How well do the paragraphs funnel the reader?

9.8.1 Initial Version

Health equity cannot exist without data equity. This pilot study will assess the extent to which a linked US Veterans Health Administration-Department of Defense data source supports subgroup (or disaggregated) studies of minority veterans. Asian Americans and Pacific Islanders are two of the fastest-growing segments of the current and future US veteran population. But their healthcare needs remain understudied. Disaggregation of health data on Asian American and Pacific Islander subgroups—a national priority made urgent by executive orders issued at the height of the COVID-19 pandemic—can reveal disparities otherwise hidden or erased when these subgroups are lumped together or included only in an "other" category. We can actively move toward data equity by leveraging military personnel records containing rich ethnicity information.

9.8.2 Revision

Despite their status as two of the fastest-growing veteran groups, little is known about the health and healthcare needs of US Asian Americans and Pacific Islanders. The COVID-19 pandemic showed how the reduction of diverse subgroups into a single racial category—or, worse, erasure by inclusion only in an "other" category—perpetuates stereotypes about Asian Americans and Pacific Islanders as "model minorities" who have few health or social needs, because if nothing is known about these subgroups, nothing can be said or done about their needs. As evidenced by executive orders issued at the pandemic's height, analyzing the specific health data of Asian American and Pacific Islander subgroups is a critical first step to prevent devastating health outcomes, eliminate health disparities, and achieve health equity. This proposed pilot study explores a novel linkage of Veterans Health Administration and Department of Defense data to support specific subgroup studies of Asian American and Pacific Islander veterans.

9.8.3 Final Version

During the COVID-19 pandemic, US Asian Americans and Pacific Islanders suffered disproportionate negative health outcomes, yet—despite the availability of adequate data—research analyses frequently ignored their experiences. In research, the two groups were often reduced into a single racial category or, worse, entirely erased from analyses by being lumped with other groups into an "other" category. This data aggregation not only unfairly hid the cost that Asian Americans and Pacific Islanders paid during the pandemic but also perpetuated stereotypes about Asian Americans and Pacific Islanders being "model minorities" who have few health or social needs, because without data, nothing was known. Such data aggregation procedures also mean that, despite Asian Americans and Pacific Islanders being two of the fastest-growing US veteran groups, little is known about variations in sociodemographic characteristics and health and healthcare needs across these subgroups. As evidenced by executive orders issued at the pandemic's height, studying the specific health data of Asian American and Pacific Islander subgroups is a critical first step to target health interventions, eliminate health disparities, and achieve health equity. This proposed pilot study explores a novel linkage of Department of Defense and Veterans Health Administration data to support specific subgroup studies of Asian Americans and Pacific Islander veterans.

Below are the three versions again, this time with annotations about the hook's emotional engagement, the question it opens, and its adherence to or breaks with principles about hooks. I did not comment on the relationship to funding organization priorities because each version addresses this in some form. After dissecting the initial sentence, I also note whether the subsequent sentences create an effective downward-facing funnel for the reader, indicating whether I think a statement is broad or narrow, *relative to the prior sentence.* Alternating funnel directions within a paragraph suggest potential issues. Ideally, a paragraph such as this leads a reader directly, with ever more specificity, to the goals of the study.

9.8.4 Annotated Initial Version

Health equity cannot exist without data equity. [*Pros*: The hook is short, with only one point. It covers broad ground, which enables a future focus on multiple issues, although nothing hints at what those issues might be. *Cons*: The hook is written as a negative statement. A rewording would be, "Health equity requires data equity." Whatever the phrasing, the hook uses jargon. The writer assumes a reviewer will know what is meant by "health equity" and "data equity." *Comment on audience*: A broad hook, which this is, often targets an audience at Level 1 or Level 2 of awareness. But jargon assumes a high level of awareness of the subject, probably Level 3. The conflicting assumptions about the reviewer's level of awareness create unwanted confusion in the hook. *Comment on emotional urgency*: This hook conveys little to no emotional urgency. Even a reader who understands what is meant by health equity and data equity would not feel moved, since the hook portrays neither of these as under threat. *Comment on question raised*: At a stretch, the question raised is whether data equity exists.] This pilot study will assess the extent to which a linked US Veterans Health Administration-Department of Defense data source supports subgroup (or disaggregated) studies of minority veterans. [*narrow*] Asian Americans and Pacific Islanders are two of the fastest-growing segments of the current and future US veteran population. [*broad*] But their healthcare needs remain understudied. [*narrow*] Disaggregation of health data on Asian American and Pacific Islander subgroups—a national priority made urgent by executive orders issued at the height of the COVID-19 pandemic—can reveal disparities otherwise hidden or erased when these subgroups are lumped together or included only in an "other" category. [*narrow*] We can actively move toward data equity by leveraging military personnel records containing rich ethnicity information. [*broad*].

9.8.5 Annotated Revision

Despite their status as two of the fastest-growing veteran groups, little is known about the health and healthcare needs of US Asian Americans and Pacific Islanders. [*Pros*: The hook introduces the population of interest. It avoids jargon, using language anyone can understand. *Cons*: The hook begins with a longer, somewhat complex (in terms of ideas) introductory phrase. The sentence wording could be reordered, so the population of interest comes first, which would improve cognitive ease: "Little is known about the health and healthcare needs of Asian Americans and Pacific Islanders, despite their status as two of the fastest growing veteran groups." *Comment on audience*: The hook here is broad, assuming an awareness of Level 1. The vocabulary used is consistent with this level. *Comment on emotional urgency*: This hook conveys some emotional urgency because it juxtaposes the rapid growth of this population group with knowing little about their health and healthcare. *Comment on question raised*: The hook implicitly raises the question of how we can learn more about this population and rectify the situation. Note that it could also raise other questions, including *why* nothing is known. Ideally, the hook only raises one question. But sometimes a writer must be content with piquing a reviewer's interest in the first sentence and rely on subsequent sentences to guide to the main issue.] The COVID-19 pandemic showed how the reduction of diverse subgroups into a single racial category—or, worse, erasure into an "other" category—perpetuates stereotypes about Asian Americans and Pacific Islanders as "model minorities" who have few health or social needs, because if nothing is known about these subgroups, nothing can be said or done about their needs. [*narrow*] As evidenced by executive orders issued at the pandemic's height, analyzing the specific health data of Asian American and Pacific Islander subgroups is a critical first step to prevent devastating health outcomes, eliminate health disparities, and achieve health equity. [*broad*] This proposed pilot study explores a novel linkage of Veterans Health Administration and Department of Defense data to support specific subgroup studies of Asian Americans and Pacific Islander veterans. [*narrow*].

9.8.6 Annotated Final Version

During the COVID-19 pandemic, US Asian Americans and Pacific Islanders suffered disproportionate negative health outcomes, yet—despite the availability of adequate data—research analyses frequently ignored their experiences. [*Pros*: The hook identifies the population of interest and the method of interest.

What was described as "health equity" in the original version is now "suffered disproportionate negative health outcomes," which anyone can understand. And this change addresses the "So what?" question, showing readers what needs to change and why they should care. *Cons*: The hook is long and contains two important pieces of information (negative health outcomes and experiences ignored in data analyses), either of which could conceivably be the focus of the study. To compensate, the writer uses sentence structure to guide to the main point, with "yet" and "despite" focusing a reader on the latter half of the sentence. There are many other ways this could be done. *Comment on audience*: The hook remains broad, assumes Level 1 awareness, and uses vocabulary consistent with this level. The wording has increased slightly in complexity but is still at a level that would be easily understood by a literate scientist. *Comment on emotional urgency*: This hook deliberately targets a reviewer's emotions. The words "pandemic," "suffered," "negative," and "ignored" develop a sense of hardship and injustice. *Comment on question raised*: The hook raises curiosity about how to remedy this problem. As in the revision, it could also raise the question of why the problem occurs. Because of this, it, again, relies on subsequent sentences to instruct the reader as to the overall purpose.] In research, the two groups were often reduced into a single racial category or, worse, entirely erased from analyses by being lumped with other groups into an "other" category. [*narrow*] This data aggregation not only unfairly hid the cost Asian Americans and Pacific Islanders paid during the pandemic but also perpetuated stereotypes about Asian Americans and Pacific Islanders being "model minorities" who have few health or social needs, because without data, nothing was known. [*narrow*] Such data procedures also mean that, despite Asian Americans and Pacific Islanders being two of the fastest-growing US veteran groups, little is known about variations in sociodemographic characteristics and health and healthcare needs across these subgroups. [*narrow*] As evidenced by executive orders issued at the pandemic's height, studying the specific health data of Asian American and Pacific Islander subgroups is a critical first step to target health interventions, eliminate health disparities, and achieve health equity. [*narrow*] This proposed pilot study explores a novel linkage of Department of Defense and Veterans Health Administration data to support specific subgroup studies of Asian Americans and Pacific Islander veterans. [*narrow*].

As this example shows, hooks benefit from editing and perfection exists only in theory. Excellent hooks abound. Their creation is limited only by a writer's time and imagination. Crafting a great hook often involves balancing brevity against the need to mesh with a reviewer's level of awareness. Consider the principles above as signposts. They stress the factors at play. Decide what benefits your proposal.

References

Hartmann, C. W. (2023). How screenwriting can help your grant writing. *Nature.*

Heath, C., & Heath, D. (2007). *Made to Stick: Why Some Ideas Survive and Others Die.* Random House.

McKee, R. (1997). *Story: Substance, Structure, Style, and the Principles of Screenwriting.* Harper Collins.

Chapter 10
Summaries

In the grant world, a funding organization or reviewer usually encounters a proposal first through a letter, abstract, or other brief summary of the main ideas. Because these types of documents are short, a writer may save them for last and spend little time on them. But first impressions count. Writing a compelling synopsis requires thought, revision, and attention to detail.

Tough funding climates only accentuate the importance of summaries. As noted in Chap. 2, Sect. 2.1, when funds are scarce, reviewers frequently have additional obligations. Fewer applications might advance to review by a full committee. Funding organizations may also place other restraints on review processes or expect proposals to address the organization's funding priorities more directly. Under these circumstances, summaries become powerful tools for reviewers and others, who lean on their brevity and comprehensiveness for understanding and when advocating for a proposal.

In my early proposal-writing days, the length of a document dictated the energy I expended on it. I put the most effort into the description of my research plans, much less into the page that described the specific aims for the study, and the least into the abstract. I thought, for example, that I could create an adequate abstract by cutting and pasting phrases and sentences from a near-final draft of the main text. I did not understand the iterative nature of building a persuasive proposal and how the same processes and principles should drive content across all sections of an application. I also did not recognize the value of summaries.

Then, I was recruited to serve on a formal grant review panel and realized their significance. Summaries are often the first sections of a grant that a reviewer reads and can sway them into a relaxed (cognitive ease) or vigilant (cognitive strain) mindset. (See Chap. 1, Sect, 1.1 and Chap. 7 for more on cognitive ease.) For busy review committee members not assigned to a particular proposal, the summaries may be the *only* parts they read. Individuals making funding decisions also rely on these documents. This awareness flipped my prior writing style on its head. In subsequent applications, I reserved time to create and repeatedly edit summaries to ensure they

C. W. Hartmann, *Grant Writing Fundamentals Made Easy*,
https://doi.org/10.1007/978-3-032-35723-6_10

gave unique expression to a proposal's most important ideas. I sometimes spent as much time on these short sections as I did on the rest of the application.

10.1 Letters

A submission process often involves at least one letter. Many funding organizations, for example, require notification of an intent to submit a proposal. Some even obligate potential applicants to receive permission before submitting a proposal. Frequently, an application also includes a cover letter. The individuals who review initial letters might be different from those who review the final proposal. But because letters are by nature short and designed to summarize the application's objectives, their messages must be clear, easy to find, and convincing.

Writing a letter requires implementing the same thoughtful process required for a longer collection of text. This means beginning by organizing the content you want a reader to remember. You may feel pressure to write something quickly because the turnaround time is fast. Sometimes you see a request for proposals only days before a letter of intent is due. These and other circumstances might drive a desire to dash something off without forethought or editing. This comes with substantial risks.

As noted elsewhere, first impressions in the grant world, just as in other areas of life, count. Any initial message to an organization, be it one to notify of an intent to submit or to inquire about the organization's interest in an idea, represents the introduction both of you as a potential grantee and of your project. Focus on the task: convincing a reader that your work aligns with priorities and should move forward.

If you have a draft of the full proposal, or even just an outline, you can use that information to build a letter. If the letter represents an initial stab at concretizing an idea, your draft may require multiple iterations. Try adhering to the same steps as when constructing an application's outline, detailed in Chap. 8, Sect. 8.1. Then, show what you write to colleagues, particularly those who are not familiar with your area, or employ AI to critique the draft. Are there gaps in logic? Can readers follow your points? Are they convinced?

The funding organization likely has predetermined review criteria for letters. These might not be explicit. But often an organization hints at what it wants in the call for letters. What do they ask applicants to include? What do they indicate as topic areas or methods they are interested in? Also look at the organization's strategic plan, its objectives, and the topics of recent awardees. Many grant writing books contain explanations and examples of standard letter content. Some organizations may not want a traditional letter format but may instead require filling in an online form. In this case, you can deduce expectations from the instructions.

Once you understand the guidelines, revisit your draft to ensure it contains every point that is expected. Think creatively. Explicitly responding to formal expectations does not mean being dull, redundant, or dry. A letter that lacks required information or makes information difficult to find will usually annoy a reader. But a letter that exceeds expectations can excite.

As with the full application, a letter should reflect the 1-3-2 principle (see Chap. 7, Sect. 7.1), beginning and ending with the most important ideas. As you craft it, recognize that bolding, underlining, or otherwise highlighting information in the middle of a sentence or paragraph is a clue that you buried significant points. Emphasis does not help reviewers remember. The reader should be able to skim the first and last sentences of each paragraph or section and understand the thrust of your argument.

Following this principle leads to a second principle for letters, which is to avoid wasting space, as most letters are expected to be succinct. Some even have page, word, or character limits. Yet many letters of inquiry or intent, even successful ones, begin with statements such as, "We are writing this letter to inquire whether your organization might be willing to fund…" or, "This is a letter of intent to submit a proposal for…" They write about what they are doing. But these days, with electronic submissions, letters do not physically land on someone's desk in an envelope. The content is not a surprise. The first lines of a letter should, therefore, present the hook and whatever other information you believe will best support your case (see Chap. 9 for more on hooks).

In the first sentence, can you think outside the standard box and touch a reader's emotions? Can your letter open a question in a reader's mind about how the world would change if this application were funded? How does this work relate to the organization's current concerns? Instead of beginning an application to a multinational telecommunication corporation's foundation with, "We are writing to request $500,000 to improve internet access for rural inhabitants of our county," modify this to be more specific: "The $500,000 we request in our application will enable over 6,000 families to benefit from a novel internet access program." Or this, "Our county struggles with one of the lowest rates of internet access in the country, which is why we request $500,000 to implement our innovative internet access program to support improved connectivity for over 6,000 families who would otherwise remain technologically isolated." The more specific and emotionally engaging your hook, the more memorable it is likely to be.

Another way to drive home the importance of the proposed work and make a letter stand out is to include a concise story. In a letter limited to a page or only a few text boxes, a story may not fit. Only implement this strategy if you have a compelling idea and the space to execute it. But if your proposal lends itself to writing about a success story or an urgent need, then consider devoting a few lines or a call-out box to a brief account of a concrete, specific case, making the effect on the world tangible.

A letter should also end strong. Can you relate the final statement back to the beginning hook? Can you encapsulate the need or opportunity your application addresses with a fact or anecdote? What can you include to emphasize the future positive effect of your proposed work?

The best letters promote cognitive ease by eschewing dense text. Even when faced with tight word limits, consider how to improve a reader's cognitive ease. White space between paragraphs and ideas helps a reader pause and assimilate information. Section headings or bolded phrases at the beginning of paragraphs orient and provide signposts that the letter conforms to all expectations. If, for example, a letter must include information about prior successes, the proposal idea, and the potential effect of the award, create headings for each.

Before submission, scrutinize your letter from the 30,000-foot level. What is the big picture message for the reader? Are the points easy to recognize and follow? Have you proofread carefully? Give the letter to someone outside your field and ask them to read it. (See Chap. 4, Sects. 4.4 and 4.5 for whom to approach and how to have dialogues about your work with them.) Embrace their comments to improve cognitive ease.

The effort spent on a letter generally correlates with its success. Your goal is to craft one that contains easy-to-understand, unforgettable ideas. This requires balancing precision with creativity and prioritizing both adherence to expectations and the power of emotional effect. It requires effort. But the payoff is great.

10.2 Brief Initial Summaries

Review committees usually comprise many individuals. Of these, only a few are ordinarily assigned to read an entire application. Final decisions about funding generally rest in the hands of yet a different group. Those individuals must determine who receives money based on information from the committee and a snapshot of the proposal that is frequently taken from an application's initial summaries. All this shows that documents such as abstracts and pages that describe the project's objectives or aims represent some of a grant's most influential text.

A summary acts as a sales pitch, beginning with a strong hook, as explained in Chap. 9. Evidence supporting the main ideas follows. Many grant writing books and courses teach how to craft a standard summary introduction. As with everything else, outlining enables strategic analysis of content (see Chap. 8, Sect. 8.1) and helps ensure a logical flow (see Chap. 8, Sect. 8.3).

Traditionally, summaries include background information that sets up the objectives and aims as well as information about methods, outcome evaluations, and next steps. Summaries should instill confidence that the project will succeed and clearly indicate how the work advances the funding organization's current mission. Each paragraph or section should set up what comes next. Similar to the discussion section of a journal article, nothing at the *end* of a summary should come as a surprise or as new material. This interconnected nature of a summary means it requires careful editing. Experienced grant writers therefore often think of summaries as works in progress until just before they push the button to submit.

How much text you devote to each part of a summary commonly mirrors the amount of space allotted to the topics in the proposal's main narrative sections. For example, if the data collection description is short and the study evaluation methods description is longer, a typical summary will address these topics with less and more text, respectively. But the audience for these summaries is broader than that for the main narrative and, therefore, the critical job for a summary is to hook and convince. Do not be afraid to break with convention. Consider including a vignette or story if you have a strong reason. You can also start a summary with a question and follow that with a hypothetical scenario to engage the reviewer.

As is the case with letters, avoid descriptions of what your writing does, here and elsewhere in the proposal. Do not write, "The specific aims focus on…" Simply state the aims. Change, "We found that chemical X failed to catalyze a reaction, so…" to, "Chemical X failed to catalyze a reaction, so…" Instead of, "In this study, we will investigate…," write, "We will investigate…" Doing this not only saves space but focuses a busy reviewer on what is important.

As always, adhere to the 1-3-2/2-3-1 principle (see Chap. 7, Sect. 7.1). Close with a bang. Make it memorable. Think about how to convince someone outside your field that your objectives not only deserve exploration but *require* it. Good summaries end by answering questions such as these.

- How is this proposal unique and necessary? (This points to innovation.)
- How will this proposal change the world for the better? (This relates to outcomes, significance, and funding organization priorities.)
- What guarantees that you will be successful? (This highlights your methods and team.)
- What new avenues will this work open? (This points to future opportunities.)

The final sentences deserve your best effort, because these are the last chances to hit home with a concise reason to fund an application. Avoid populating the end of a summary with snippets that did not make it farther up the paragraph or page. Think of the ending as the last notes in a symphony, the melody you want your reader to hum on their way home.

Chapter 11
Main Narrative Sections

11.1 Spin

In the world of politics, "spin" implies deviousness, a distortion of facts. But the dictionary definition is neutral. Spin, according to Merriam-Webster (2026), is "a special point of view, emphasis, or interpretation presented for the purpose of influencing opinion." In the world of grants, spin represents a guiding principle.

A proposal's primary goal is to have reviewers believe that *this* application, above others, deserves the award. Because any issue can be seen from multiple viewpoints, an application must contain both explicit and implicit messages supporting its argument. In other words, it convinces through spin.

In a brief initial summary, for example, spin should abound. But it also applies to the main narrative sections. Everywhere, the effect of successfully completing the project should be evident. Describing how the work will change the world rests not only on facts. *How* you present evidence, even contradictory evidence, matters. If information is left out or open to multiple interpretations, a reviewer draws their own conclusions. Instead, guide a reader to logical, well-supported positions.

Exercise: Spin a Sentence

Imagine you work for a nonprofit hiking trail association. You will apply to a national conservation group for money to support a summer youth internship program. What is your first sentence? Say it aloud or write it down before reading further. Your sentence reflects what you think will sway reviewers. That is your special point of view. Your spin.

Here are a few examples, each with a different viewpoint.

A. In recent years, youth from disadvantaged neighborhoods have had less access to outdoor spaces than ever before.

B. Research shows that children need to spend time outdoors to develop a lasting affinity for nature.

C. W. Hartmann, *Grant Writing Fundamentals Made Easy*,
https://doi.org/10.1007/978-3-032-35723-6_11

C. Access to the outdoors should be a national right.

Many other sentences about the same topic are possible. The key to successful grant writing is to be explicit with yourself about what you want your reader to believe and, when appropriate, spin your factually supported position accordingly.

11.1.1 When to Spin

Below are five cases in which spin is critical.

1. You anticipate your ideas represent new ground for reviewers.
2. You anticipate reviewers' resistance.
3. You are afraid reviewers will lose your point.
4. There are multiple perspectives on an issue.
5. You want to pound home your message.

11.1.2 How to Spin

Stick with facts and specifics. Avoid vague and unsupported statements. Look at these two sentences.

A. It is important to address the high rates of cervical cancer in the incarcerated population.
B. Women in the criminal justice system have cervical cancer at a four to five times higher rate than nonincarcerated women.

You may not recognize B as spin. But leading with that message is a choice. A proposal on this topic could have begun by stating that there are one million incarcerated women in the US or that fewer than half the incarcerated women who are screened for cervical cancer get access to the recommended follow-up. But the writer of B wants to emphasize the high rates, perhaps to tap into reviewers' subconscious fears about cancer. Or maybe the writer thought it best to stick with the relatively neutral ground of rates before diving into who is incarcerated and issues driving incarcerated individuals' low access.

You might believe I credit proposal authors with too much forethought. Does a good writer wonder what sentence leads best? Yes. Many spend time rewriting and reordering their executive summaries, specific aims pages, and other overviews, particularly the first sentences and paragraph.

Present opposing views; then make them support your point. Reviewers may know as much or more about a subject as you do. Avoid any temptation to leave out perspectives that offer a counterpoint to your argument. Instead, create space for opposition, preferably in the middle of a paragraph or section. Sandwich this information between facts that support your case. (See Chap. 7, Sect. 7.1 for more on why to place less important information between more important points.)

Look at this paragraph from a publicly available grant about investigating an intervention to improve incarcerated women's health literacy to help prevent cervical cancer (National Cancer Institute, n.d., p. 8).

> We operationalized the definition of health literacy so broadly, in part because of grounding in the literature (e.g., IOM [Institute of Medicine] report), but also because such an operationalization would allow us to develop an effective intervention tailored specifically to our population and [be] responsive to findings from our preliminary studies. We realize there is substantial debate in the field of health literacy, with initial definitions of health literacy as reading, writing, and deciphering medical labels. The IOM report highlighted the need, however, to move beyond knowledge and focus on people's ability to act upon that knowledge, which we feel encompasses their beliefs about health, self-efficacy, and confidence in navigating health systems. Thus, our conception of the proposed intervention is one that focuses on "interactive health literacy," where we impart both knowledge and skills.

Do you notice how the writer sandwiched the issue of "substantial debate" between the pillars of the proposal's own argument? The author strengthened their case by clarifying that they were familiar with debates in the field and by using those issues to focus reviewers on why this application's position is correct. That is spin.

Use compelling language. Facts are compelling. Consider how fact-driven sentences in your proposal are and whether they support statements about effects. Continuing with the same health literacy and cervical cancer proposal, what facts and effects can you find in the following two sentences taken from the first paragraph of that application's specific aims page? "The one million women incarcerated in the US—95% of whom will return to their communities—are mostly poor, racial/ethnic minorities with long histories of abuse, mental health problems, drug use, and STIs [sexually transmitted infections]. These complex factors exacerbate their risk for cervical cancer, as well as create barriers to follow-up health care" (National Cancer Institute, n.d., p. 6). I count eight facts and two effects in two sentences. That is a goal worth shooting for.

Organize your messages logically. Avoid skipping around. Create a logical flow that guides readers to a perspective on the narrative you present (see Chap. 8, Sect. 8.3). The same cervical cancer proposal's specific aims page first paragraph, reduced by me to summary bullets, looks like this.

- Incarcerated women get a lot of cancer, but the reason for this is understudied.
- The US has many incarcerated women, most of whom have lived through many hardships.
- The hardships put these women at risk for both cancer and lack of follow-up care.
- The investigators found health literacy plays a role in these two things.
- So we must address health literacy.

Another writer could have organized differently or presented alternative information. That is the point. There are multiple ways to write a grant about the same subject matter. As long as you present material logically, accurately, and comprehensively, you can create compelling spin about *your* viewpoint.

Remember, spin is a four-letter word to embrace with all its complex nuances. It represents an opportunity and an advantage. Understanding and employing it gives you an edge over your competition.

11.2 Introductions

A proposal's narrative often includes a shorter introduction. These vary in length. Funding organizations have assorted names for this part, including specific aims, project summary, program plan, and case for support. It serves as a guide for what comes next and supports the grant's objectives. By the time a reader reaches those objectives, nothing (topic or methods) should come as a surprise. Leave details until later in the application. But all high-level issues referenced by the objectives should be addressed before the reader gets to them.

Here is an example from an online grant repository; it is the introduction to the narrative section from a successful proposal submitted by the Alexandria Archive Institute for an Infrastructure and Capacity Building Challenge Grant from the US National Endowment for the Humanities. (See Chap. 4, Sect. 4.2 for what to look for when dissecting grant examples.) There are 8 sentences in total.

> The Alexandria Archive Institute (AAI) seeks a National Endowment for the Humanities Infrastructure and Capacity Building Challenge Grant for a project with the following elements: (1) expansion of our core archaeological data publishing and archiving services; (2) development of a data literacy program for broader public education; and (3) establishment of a consortium of museum, library, and other institutional sponsors to sustain open access to archaeological data into the future. The challenges inherent in understanding and using digital data are as intellectually demanding as any other humanistic research endeavor. Confronting these challenges requires dependable institutional and financial support. The AAI has a 15-year record of success publishing major data data sets, books, and peer-reviewed articles. The AAI's staff holds leadership positions in scholarly societies, policy-making committees, and granting programs, advocating change in professional attitudes toward data. In 2013, the White House celebrated our contributions with a "Champion of Change Award," and we subsequently earned awards from the digital library and archaeological research communities. Even with these tremendous strides, our operations as an independent nonprofit organization rely on tenuous, high-risk grant support. To build a stronger foundation for continuity and growth, our Challenge Grant project will strengthen and diversify broader community engagement and institutional partnerships. (National Endowment for the Humanities, n.d., p. 2)

Below, after each original sentence, I present an alternative. The original version, obviously, convinced reviewers. My alternative is not necessarily better. I present alternatives to showcase principles for writing introductions. I challenge you to think of your own alternatives and justifications for your decisions before looking at mine. I have my viewpoint—you have your own. Speak your thoughts aloud or write them down. The more you participate, the more you will learn about your own writing style.

11.2.1 First Sentence

"The Alexandria Archive Institute (AAI) seeks a National Endowment for the Humanities Infrastructure and Capacity Building Challenge Grant for a project with the following elements: (1) expansion of our core archaeological data publishing and archiving services; (2) development of a data literacy program for broader public education; and (3) establishment of a consortium of museum, library, and other institutional sponsors to sustain open access to archaeological data into the future." [In the application, this long sentence was a stand-alone paragraph.]

What do you think? How would you revise this sentence and why? Take a moment to say your own ideas aloud or write them down.

An alternative: I like the original sentence, particularly the way it homes in on what the writers seek funding for. But the first part of the sentence is not necessary, since a reviewer already knows what kind of grant they are reviewing. Instead, a writer could focus on *why* this project is important, putting the project in context. I extrapolated from what is publicly available on the AAI's website. I propose beginning with two sentences such as this: "The Alexandria Archive Institute (AAI) fills a unique and critical need by preserving the world's archaeological heritage and opening it up to all. The current project helps execute this mission by (1) expanding our core archaeological data publishing and archiving services; (2) developing a data literacy program for broader public education; and (3) establishing a consortium of museum, library, and other institutional sponsors to sustain open access to archaeological data into the future."

11.2.2 Second Sentence

"The challenges inherent in understanding and using digital data are as intellectually demanding as any other humanistic research endeavor."

What do you think? Say your own ideas aloud or write them down.

An alternative: This sentence "tells" a reader something they should believe instead of "showing" them evidence for why a position or statement is true. (See Chap. 7, Sect. 7.5 on the importance of showing.) Why should a reviewer believe that understanding and using digital data are difficult? Instead, I suggest writing about something relevant and more tangible, such as how much data AAI deals with on an annual basis. This could be something such as, "AAI collects and analyzes ___ [amount] of data annually, resulting in ___ [number] of publications per year." This sentence uses facts to underscore the demanding nature of AAI's work. A different, potentially more memorable approach would be to employ an analogy, such as, "AAI collects and analyzes ___ [amount] of data annually, meaning that if one gigabyte [or terabyte] of data were the equivalent of a city block, every year AAI deals with data about the size of ___ [Baltimore/Berlin/Beijing]."

11.2.3 Third Sentence

"Confronting these challenges requires dependable institutional and financial support."

What do you think? Say your own ideas aloud or write them down.

An alternative: As a follow-up to a fact-based prior sentence, I like this. I do not have any suggested changes, except to align this sentence with the prior one, as in, "Confronting the challenges inherent in AAI's work requires dependable institutional and financial support."

11.2.4 Fourth Sentence

"The AAI has a 15-year record of success publishing major data data sets, books, and peer-reviewed articles."

What do you think? Say your own ideas aloud or write them down.

An alternative: I am not clear how this relates to the prior sentence. I also do not understand what a "major data data set" is. I first thought the double use of "data" was a typo and then realized it might mean a data set that is based on large data. With these two things in mind, I would change the sentence to something like, "The AAI has a 15-year history of securing institutional and financial resources that have enabled a successful publishing record including ___ [here I would list numbers instead of simply nouns, such as *how many* data sets, books, articles, etc.]"

11.2.5 Fifth Sentence

"The AAI's staff holds leadership positions in scholarly societies, policy-making committees, and granting programs, advocating change in professional attitudes towards data."

What do you think? Say your own ideas aloud or write them down.

An alternative: The narrative thread, given my change above, now leads to a plausible continuation of the list of AAI accomplishments to date. This creates an opportunity for spin (see Sect. 11.1), with a sentence such as this: "Undergirding this success is AAI's ability to advocate for change in professional attitudes toward data, which AAI enables through AAI staff holding leadership positions in scholarly societies, policy-making committees, and granting programs."

11.2.6 Sixth Sentence

"In 2013, the White House celebrated our contributions with a 'Champion of Change Award', and we subsequently earned awards from the digital library and archaeological research communities."

What do you think? Say your own ideas aloud or write them down.

An alternative: The sentence is fine. But it makes two points that could be related to each other. It could also flow more smoothly with the narrative. One alternative is the following: "In recognition of its numerous achievements, AAI received the White House 2013 'Champion of Change Award' and subsequent awards from the digital library and archaeological research communities."

11.2.7 Seventh Sentence

"Even with these tremendous strides, our operations as an independent non-profit organization rely on tenuous, high-risk grant support."

What do you think? Say your own ideas aloud or write them down.

An alternative: I like the point of this sentence. But I do not like the word "strides," which implies AAI is still on its way, as opposed to already having achieved success. Here is an option: "AAI's significant accomplishments belie the fact that its operations as an independent nonprofit organization rely on tenuous, high-risk grant support."

11.2.8 Final Sentence

"To build a stronger foundation for continuity and growth, our Challenge Grant project will strengthen and diversify broader community engagement and institutional partnerships."

What do you think? Say your own ideas aloud or write them down.

An alternative: This is a strong ending. But I might reverse the order, so it ends with the reason for the grant (the why), instead of the what. This is an individual decision. A revised final sentence might look like this: "This Challenge Grant project will strengthen and diversify AAI's broader community engagement and institutional partnerships, establishing a stronger foundation for continuity and continued growth."

How do you feel after critically appraising a well-written, successful application? Were your changes similar to or different from mine? Critically assessing funded grants helps you adopt what you like and identify what you could improve about your own writing.

11.3 Background Information

The first part of a proposal's main narrative section often introduces foundational information. This section (called the introduction, statement of need, problem section, background section, etc.) provides evidence that grounds the application's specific aims, including methods and, potentially, the environment or team. It convinces readers that the project will accomplish its goals. Successful sections often do the following.

They adhere to the proposal's overarching organization. The background-providing section should present material in the same order as the rest of the application. If a proposal argues that planting more trees along streets will help with noise pollution, promote safer driving habits, and have environmental benefits, this section should address the elements in that order. It seems like an easy principle to follow. But many background-providing sections jump around, presumably following the order in which it was easiest to write them. Instead, the section's logic should mirror that of any initial summary (executive summary, cover letter, or abstract). If there are no preceding sections and the proposal format requires diving immediately into supporting evidence, the evidence can begin with a brief statement that hooks the reader and lays a logical foundation.

They funnel the reader. Classic organization involves funneling from broad to increasingly narrower topics and ending on the crucial point (see Chap. 8, Sect. 8.3). Most proposals follow this or similar approaches. When doing this, each heading should address a question that arises from the proposal's arguments. Each application has its own set of questions. Answering these rests a premise on solid ground.

They cover all relevant topics. The background-providing section should cover every premise in a proposal, from main issue to population, conceptual framework to methods, and more. Reviewers expect this section to be comprehensive. If you find relevant background material in subsequent sections, move it up to this section. Later sections may repeat key points. But they should not raise new ones.

They include known controversies and explain how these affect the proposal. One important aspect of background-providing sections is thoroughness. This includes embracing controversies in the field. To return to the tree planting example, if there is a known problem of pests killing the usual types of street-lining trees, address this directly by describing the problem and explaining how you will overcome it by, for example, planting a type of tree known to be pest resistant. If a similar group recently started a bush-planting campaign in the community, demonstrate how trees will complement the existing bushes or how trees and bushes will be planted on separate blocks. Never assume reviewers are ignorant of a controversy. Reviewers appreciate grants that explain potential obstacles and spell out proposed plans. This is the mark of an honest, thoughtful, and solution-oriented applicant.

The authors outline first (see Sect. 8.1). Gaps in logic stand out particularly strongly in background-providing sections because these contain more detail than any earlier summaries. If a key point is missing or the logic does not flow well, reviewers are much more likely to notice. Outlines help catch and avoid such issues.

Section headings should provide meaningful information. Headings (or first sentences of paragraphs if headings are not possible) should not only describe subsequent content but also emphasize the urgency or importance of the issue. To continue with the tree-lined streets example, the heading for the background about noise pollution could be descriptive, such as, "Roadside trees and noise pollution." But a more meaningful heading might be, "Roadside trees represent a cost-effective way to reduce noise pollution," or, "Cities with roadside trees have significantly less noise pollution." Both latter options indicate that data support the connection. They also foreshadow what data will be presented: cost-effectiveness data in the first and magnitude of the effect in the second.

They include graphics where relevant (see Sect. 11.7). If allowed, graphics provide a valuable opportunity to display a large amount of material in a relatively small space. Create a figure or table where a visual display helps the reader. The final version of the proposal might not need all the graphics you create. But the process of creating a figure or table can, in and of itself, help you focus on the most relevant content, which can aid you in writing text more pertinent to the central issue.

Grant writers may use AI software to help with conducting an initial literature review, summarizing articles, or diving deeper into topics. Some writers use it for much more than that. AI software can provide timesaving help and useful preliminary directions. It can also supply a valuable assessment of a draft. Before enlisting the help of AI, check whether the funding organization has conditions around or prohibitions against its use. (See Chap. 1, Sect. 1.3 for more on AI use in grant writing.)

11.4 Plans and Methods for Achieving Objectives

The section or sections that describe plans and methods for achieving objectives require special attention. Most commonly, these sections are called the following: research plan, narrative, objectives, evaluation plan, intellectual rationale, program design, work plan, methods, or methodology. Each funding organization uses specific terminology and has unique requirements. Reviewers usually judge proposals on some variant of the rigor and feasibility of the approaches explained in these sections.

Up to this point in a proposal's narrative, reviewers do not know much about project design or execution. These sections dive into detail, clearly outlining plans that cover both the how and the why of each step. Many books and websites about grant writing describe the standard parts of this type of section. Components include the goals and objectives for the work; specific, measurable outcomes; and comprehensive implementation and evaluation plans. But in addition to adhering to these standard expectations, these sections must also successfully persuade.

A writer must match content to known review criteria (see Chap. 4, Sect. 4.3). This is easiest to do at the outline stage, by shifting content to create a flow that pairs with how reviewers will need material. In the text writing stage, you can use wording from the criteria, as appropriate, in headings and first or last sentences to serve as signposts. A reviewer searching for information on feasibility may benefit from a heading such as, "Feasibility of our approach is assured by continual involvement of key stakeholders." After this, you can specify how you will gather and use input from stakeholders to ensure that the intervention works. If reviewers must assess goals separately from objectives, these two components should have separate headings or, at least, separate paragraphs. If reviewers are instructed to evaluate the *clarity* of a proposal's methods, the proposal can employ headings that summarize a method, along with text that outlines the consecutive steps and details. If each activity requires a milestone, perhaps create a table listing activities, dates, and milestones. Above all, avoid making a reviewer dig.

Embracing the principles of cognitive ease (see Chap. 1, Sect. 1.1 and Chap. 7 for more on cognitive ease) also means extrapolating *beyond* explicit review criteria. A successful plans and methods section addresses a reviewer's *implicit* questions. The explicit and implicit interact, meaning a strong application addresses both.

Here are examples of implicit questions to which a reviewer might unconsciously search for answers.

Why are these plans the best possible ones for the stated objectives? A proposal's objectives can conceivably be achieved using various methods. Reviewers may think of numerous ways they would approach the same problem. The ideas that come to their minds may not be the ones you propose. Yet you chose your plans for good reasons. For every major step, therefore, consider briefly outlining the main alternatives. Then, explain why your choice is better. What data or experience supports your decision? Convince a reviewer that you understand all aspects of the issue and selected wisely.

Never assume reviewers will accept things as written because they make sense to you. Avoid trying to save space by jumping over any intellectual back-and-forth that preceded the final choice. Reviewers appreciate the thoroughness implied by a succinct discussion of alternatives. They are more likely to accept a plan that does not match their own vision if their ideas were considered but set aside for clearly stated and logically argued reasons.

What risks are entailed, and how are they anticipated? Risks are inherent in any undertaking. They might exist in theory or in fact. They can be intellectual or physical. They may apply currently or only in the future. Whatever the case, you must anticipate and address them.

Reassure reviewers that you have procedures for tackling potential obstacles. Some successful proposals do this by adding periodic subsections that directly address possible risks, limitations, and ways to resolve these. A single subsection on risks and limitations can also come near the end of the entire plan/method-focused section. Alternatively, a table or logic model (see Chap. 8, Sect. 8.5) often works well for proposals with many activities and milestones, with columns for potential risks and their mitigation strategies.

How do the plans account for the larger context? Context has to do with biological, physical, or social environments. And, for an exploratory grant focused on a specific scientific idea or method, it could refer to something purely intellectual, such as advancing the state of knowledge in a field. The larger context for a proposal depends on the type of work in question, for example, community-focused ideas versus those directed at advancing bench science; exploratory anthropological research versus disease prevention; and funding to build housing versus that supporting space exploration.

Regardless of the focus, context interacts with plans. Intellectual debates affect how an idea proceeds. Environments affect how, when, and where methods have the greatest impact. Reviewers understand this. So whenever appropriate, plans should state how and why the broader context will be accounted for and, if it increases risk or imposes limits, what plans exist to reduce or eliminate potential negative effects.

What makes this team the right one to do this work? Proposals usually require space devoted to a team's credentials. This may be part of the plan-focused section or a different part. But a reviewer also gleans information about the team throughout the application. If answers to the above questions are clearly visible, a reviewer senses thoroughness, attention to detail, and strong project management skills. In other words, if the text explicitly addresses implicit questions, a reviewer will have faith that the group that wrote the application can complete the proposed project within the stated timeframe.

Many grants fail to move beyond explicit assumptions and the standard components outlined in application instructions or review criteria. Yet reviewers always judge a proposal for both what it does and what it fails to do, what it says and what it fails to say. An application might comply with instructions but fail to explain alternatives. It might detail plans but ignore potential risks. A project could seem to work on paper, but if the application does not illustrate how it will work in the real world, reviewers may have questions.

A reviewer should finish a section on plans and methods feeling confident that what is described will not only result in the application's objectives being met but that the plans and methods will ensure precision and rigor within the time proposed. Try as they might, they should not be able to conjure a scenario in which the proposal will not succeed. They may find fault with small portions. But fatal flaws should be absent.

Text that generates this kind of reaction requires dedication to moving beyond standard and stated expectations. It requires employing a strategy that anticipates concerns, both explicit and implicit, and explicitly addresses them.

11.5 Describing Innovation

Many funding organizations want a narrative section that indicates how an idea stands out. What is the proposal's contribution to the field, a community, science, or the world? This section is called different things depending on the funding organization: at the US National Institutes of Health, it is called "Innovation;" at the US Department of Veterans Affairs, "significance;" and at the US National Science Foundation, "broader impacts." I will call it the innovation section. If you find it difficult to write, you are not alone. Even highly seasoned grant writers struggle because this section either raises doubts about the application's worthiness or hammers home the significance of the work.

Regard this section as a gift. It may be the only section that directly addresses a scored review criterion in only one or a few paragraphs. Its brevity is a reason many people battle with writing it. Concise, compelling writing takes time. But succinct prose also accentuates strengths.

To write convincingly, gather successful examples and analyze what you like and do not like about them (see Chap. 4, Sect. 4.2). Find awarded proposals online that were submitted to the same or similar funding organizations. Ask colleagues, mentors, and friends for their funded applications. Locate the names of prior years' awardees and reach out to them. Not everyone will share their grant. But some will.

When you read funded proposals' innovation sections, take note of what moves you. What do you like and what turns you off? In what context do writers place their ideas? How do they use statistics, existing literature, or other studies? Do they draw analogies or anticipate potential reviewer concerns? Are their sentences long or short? Do they employ bullets or only text? Whether you are an experienced grant writer or writing your first proposal, you can always learn from reading someone else's work, especially when drafting a section that is difficult to write well.

Once you have examples, outline before writing (see Chap. 8, Sect. 8.1). Play with beginnings and endings for the section, keeping the 1-3-2/2-3-1 principle in mind (see Chap. 7, Sect. 7.1). An outline is easy to shop around for feedback from colleagues and others. You can also enlist AI to help refine a draft.

Focus on what makes your project special. Reviewers assume you are the expert on your subject. This section should reflect that knowledge. What is novel or unique, how and where does the work push the envelope, and what advantages does it have over what has been done before? Why do you have passion for this subject? What are the competing ideas and why is yours better?

As you do this, think big. Move beyond your comfort zone while avoiding the curse of knowledge (see Chap. 7, Sect. 7.2). Your reviewers are intelligent, perceptive individuals likely to come from various disciplines. If your arguments demand too much insider knowledge, you may not convince anyone. Look at how other proposals walk the line of sounding authoritative without relying on jargon (see Chap. 7, Sect. 7.3) or unexpressed assumptions. Often, placing your work within a broader context will help. Describe what is already known or has been done. Highlight why your goals are important.

Ask others to look at an outline or draft text (see Chap. 4, Sect. 4.4). Does it make sense to them? Can they understand it without background? Does it flow well? If nothing else, ask what sentence was most persuasive. Examine whether that sentence is at the beginning or end of a paragraph or buried in the middle (where people may forget it). Next, ask them for the weakest argument. Do people agree on the weak point? Can you cut it and replace it with something else? Or should it be placed in a different context? Use a prereview as an opportunity to determine what makes your proposal special in the eyes of those who are not directly invested in its success. Bring this section, or an outline of it, to your next party, lunch, or sports event. Pass it among attendees. You might be surprised by what you learn about how your ideas are received.

Above all, start early and revise continually (see Chap. 3, Sect. 3.3). As with everything else in grant writing, this section benefits from an iterative approach. Draft, get feedback, edit, and then put it away for a bit. When you return to it, edit with a critical, distanced eye. Repeat this cycle as often as you have time for. Never assume convincing innovation sections from successful proposals were slapped together in an afternoon. The better you thought they were, the more likely the writers took time to craft and revise them.

In the end, the innovation section represents only one criterion by which a proposal is evaluated. But it does something other sections do not—it highlights your work concisely within a frame of your own choosing. It is up to you to select what emphasizes your proposal's unique and valuable aspects in their best light.

11.6 Explaining the Unusual

Grant awards are prestigious to the extent they are selective. A proposal is likely to compete with many other applications for limited slots. Making your project stand out from the crowd is critical. But what if your proposal already stands out for reasons that may not, initially, seem in your favor?

As in the case of controversies, it is best to address any unexpected aspects directly. Reviewers understand that ideas come in diverse packages. Individual and organizational circumstances vary. But most successful applications contain certain elements: they are founded on what is already known, employ strong methods, point to a documented history of success, and rely on a well-organized team. When an application contains unusual elements, particularly those that contrast with reviewers' expectations, the proposal needs to acknowledge these elements and include clear, logical reasons for why divergence from the norm constitutes an advantage.

Consider the analogous situation of a job interview. Interviewers often ask applicants to talk about their "greatest weakness." Savvy interviewees understand how to flip this question to highlight their strengths, as in, "One of my weaknesses is my focus on deadlines. In the past, this meant I sometimes ignored circumstances beyond the task at hand that I later realized I should have paid attention to. But I learned from my mistakes and now implement a system that holds me accountable for deadlines *and* the entire process in which deadline completion takes place. This means I now monitor both trees *and* forest. It has improved my products while keeping me on task and on time."

For proposals that contain unusual elements, it helps to develop a similarly coherent narrative that ties everything together, including the differences. Find a common thread and weave it through every part. Every proposal tells a story.

In college, I was a German literature major and spent part of my junior year in Nepal. After graduating, I lived for nine years in Japan teaching English. When studying for my PhD, I decided to conduct my dissertation research on interdependent and independent sense of self in rural Japan. After that, my initial academic job was in a department of health policy where I conducted studies on issues related to the US health system, particularly safety. I gradually focused my research on nursing homes and wrote a mentored award for career development about improving patient safety through improving the teamwork culture of nursing home staff. This was my first large grant application. My career path at that point was, to say the least, winding.

For many people in my field, their undergraduate degree was linked to what they later pursued. Most also proceeded quickly from undergraduate to graduate or medical school. My German literature major and study abroad in Nepal was unusual. The nine-year gap in Japan was also an anomaly. In addition, my lack of formal postdoctoral training stood out. For the mentored career development proposal, I needed to market my unexpected history as a strength.

I used the theme of "culture" to tie the disparate aspects together: culture of different countries (Germany, Nepal, and Japan), culture related to psychology (dissertation), culture within a health system (safety), and culture within a nursing home (the proposal). Believe me, my story did not feel connected like this as I lived it. But it made sense when I wrote it because I left out what did not matter and crafted a theme around what did.

This leads to another principle: leave out irrelevant aspects unless doing so raises questions. If you worked for three years after college at a poetry magazine and are now a PhD-trained biochemist applying for a mentored career development award, start the narrative of your career with graduate school. No one will notice because not discussing what happened before your terminal degree is normal. But imagine that *after* getting your PhD in biochemistry, your first job was three years as a poetry magazine editor. If you leave this out of your timeline, reviewers may notice the gap, which raises questions. But including it draws attention to a puzzling oddity. In a case such as this, find a way to underscore how poetry editing helped in your current career. Have you published more scientific articles than your peers because you are better at writing? Did the awareness of detail you learned through editing poetry benefit you as you worked with microbes?

As another example, imagine you are a physician with a general internal medicine background. The thrust of your team's research to date has been in studying physician burnout. But you now want to switch topics and investigate experiences of clinicians working in oncology. Find a link between the two that supports the change. Does the new research employ related methods or address analogous issues? Can you tell a story about when oncology hooked you and connect that to the research you were doing at the time? Is there overlap in your collaborative team to highlight as a strength?

Going back to the tree planting example from Sect. 11.3, what if your tree-planting organization unexpectedly lost a major funding source due to unavoidable circumstances and the current proposal is written to fill the shortfall? An unexplained withdrawal of support looks bad. Highlighting past work will raise the question of why you need to approach a new funding organization and whether the loss of prior funding was due to an *avoidable* failure. One technique under these circumstances would be to follow the 1-3-2/2-3-1 principle (Chap. 7, Sect. 7.1). Sandwich the loss of funding as a "3" between a positive "1" and a "2." In the following example, the theme tying these together is having an excellent record of success.

1 = Our organization has planted and maintained thousands of trees, resulting in high community satisfaction, significantly lower noise levels, and fewer traffic accidents.
3 = Our prior funding from ABC Organization grew by $15,000 per year over the past ten years, due to our success record, leaving us in a strong position to now leverage new funding sources to the community's advantage.
2 = Supported by our community partners and based on our outstanding record, this proposal highlights growth opportunities for both our organization and our community.

There are many ways to package a discrepancy. Avoid shoving it under the rug. Different does not mean bad. It can make your application stand out. But difference without explanation leaves the door open for interpretations that may not be favorable. Create a logical flow with enough detail to be credible. Avoid taking a defensive posture. Instead, concentrate on controlling the narrative in a way that puts the ideas in the best light possible.

I have seen reviewers both reject and respond enthusiastically to proposals with unusual elements. The difference was whether the applicant tied things together logically. Always remember your primary audience is a smart and thoughtful group of busy people who generally start the review process by giving an applicant the benefit of the doubt. Capitalize on their beneficence. If your proposal contains deviations from the norm, invest the time to explain how this benefits you, the project, and the funding organization.

11.7 Figures and Tables

In the main narrative sections, space is at a premium. This leads, naturally, to the question of whether a graphic is worth the room it consumes. The answer is…it depends.

A good figure or table delivers content in a way text never can. It focuses the reader on crucial details or provides a depiction of an otherwise opaque subject. It clarifies associations, explicates data, offers an overview, or draws connections between items. It can tell a story, relating abstract numbers to points a reviewer or funding organization cares about. You might want people to remember a single statistic that would otherwise be overlooked. Or you may need to present results of a large analysis. Whatever the case, good figures and tables are memorable. In contrast, poor ones confuse, distract, and waste reviewer time. So how do you make good ones?

Invest time. Avoid rushing something together. Any initial idea, graphic, or representation usually requires editing. Often, the first version makes sense to the person who created it but not to outsiders. An initial draft does not always expose the principal elements. Conversely, as you revise the proposal's narrative, even a well-depicted graphic can become less important over time and may need to be cut.

If you are good at software, begin electronically. If not, begin on paper. Using AI can be a valuable and time-saving initial step. You can ask it to suggest potential figure or table types and advice on what to include, how to display information, and what to highlight. If you have a conversation with it about an idea, it can help create a visual metaphor. But be careful when and how you use it, always deferring to the funding organization's restrictions, if any, on AI's use (see Chap. 1, Sect. 1.3).

Many successful grant writers initially create multiple versions of a graphic to avoid the trap of liking what you see because you have it, not because it tells the best story. A figure or table does not have to be gorgeous. But it must convey a message. It must be worth *more* than the text space it occupies. So take care to make it the best it can be.

Which to use, figure or table? Not everyone is comfortable with making a figure. A table often seems easier to construct. But readers find bar graphs, line graphs, and component displays (such as pie charts or donut charts) easier to skim than a table. Consider using them when you can. Some information also simply demands a figure, such as logic models, organizational charts, and conceptual frameworks.

When presenting data, however, tables often seem a reasonable choice. But dense tables overwhelm a reader, particularly if the meaning is not readily identifiable. Balance what you want to include against what a reviewer needs. Your pilot study data analysis may have used many variables. But does the reviewer require the results for all of them? You may have a table from a presentation or a manuscript and feel tempted to reuse it. But are all the data relevant to the application?

Organize information logically. In English, we read from left to right and top to bottom. Reviewers will therefore read figures and tables the same way. Place important material accordingly. Bolding or coloring will not draw a reader's eye to the bottom right corner first. Instead, position material with awareness of the order in which reviewers will see it.

Whether you choose a figure or table, use neutral colors for backgrounds and data displays and then layer emphasis on top of this. Color and shading, bolding, larger font, clustering, varying shapes or styles, and call-out boxes or bubbles are some ways of distinguishing numbers, text, and shapes to draw attention to critical details.

Variation in figure and table placement also increases reader engagement. Some figures or tables can span the width of a page. Others can be left or right justified with text wrapped around them on the non-margin side. When doing this, avoid creating a difficult reading environment. Do not force a reviewer to read only a few words per line because a figure or table is not quite as wide as a page. Instead, make such a figure or table stand on its own, with text only above and below it. Also, do not make a reader jump *across* a figure or table to read each line of text (that is, avoid center justification with text wrapped around *both* sides of a figure or table).

Avoid shortcuts. If you have a figure or table from a published paper, you may think of taking a quick screenshot and dropping that into a proposal. But from the perspective of a reviewer, these types of easy insertions usually result in fuzzy and mis-sized text, making the graphic difficult to read. It is better to create a new figure or table in a software application that will copy well as a picture. Creating these from scratch also enables you to strip away nonessential information and convey only the points that support your argument. Squash the desire to take the easy route. It only means easy for you, not the reviewer.

And always avoid inserting minuscule text in your figure or table to save space. The guidelines for federal grant applications in the US indicate a minimum size of nine-point font. Adhere to the rules because reviewers expect and appreciate being able to read without having to zoom in or unearth a magnifying glass.

Figures and tables must convey meaning by themselves. Every graphic must be comprehensible and elucidating *without any accompanying text.* Why? Because a reviewer may not read your text. They might jump directly to the graphic. And if they do not understand that, or if it confuses them, they may react with annoyance. Raise your hand if you want an annoyed reviewer. Thought so.

Check others' understanding of a graphic. Run drafts by colleagues who are not familiar with your work. This is an important step. What speaks volumes to you must also speak volumes to a reviewer. So let someone outside your field, someone who has not read your application, look at a figure or table and tell you what they think it means. Avoid the temptation to explain or defend yourself or the graphic if they talk about things they do not understand. You cannot explain or defend yourself to a reviewer. Instead, take careful notes.

Use what works. Ensure the final product is of high quality. If you have administrative help with the visual formatting aspects, enjoy the support. But early in a career, one must often fend for oneself. JPEG, PNG, or SVG file images of figures usually work well. A figure or table created in PowerPoint often copies cleanly. You can also create tables directly in Word or Pages. Search online for instructions if you are unfamiliar with how to best copy, resize, or format figures or tables when inserting them into documents.

Benefit from the pause graphics enable. Figures and tables do more than display information. They interrupt the flow of text, breaking up the visual impression of a page and creating an intermission for the reader. A reviewer who analyzes a graphic engages a different part of their brain. They slow down. If the visual is clear and tells a story, this feels gratifying.

Figures 11.1, 11.2, 11.3, 11.4, 11.5, 11.6, 11.7, 11.8, 11.9, 11.10 and 11.11 are examples of figures and tables. They are not perfect. You may regularly design more beautiful graphics. I include a "sufficient" version and at least one "better" version. The sufficient ones mimic what I regularly see in journals and grant applications. The better versions showcase various methods to focus a reader on a point. As you dissect the examples, think about what helps you understand (or not) each of them. What do you like? What would you improve?

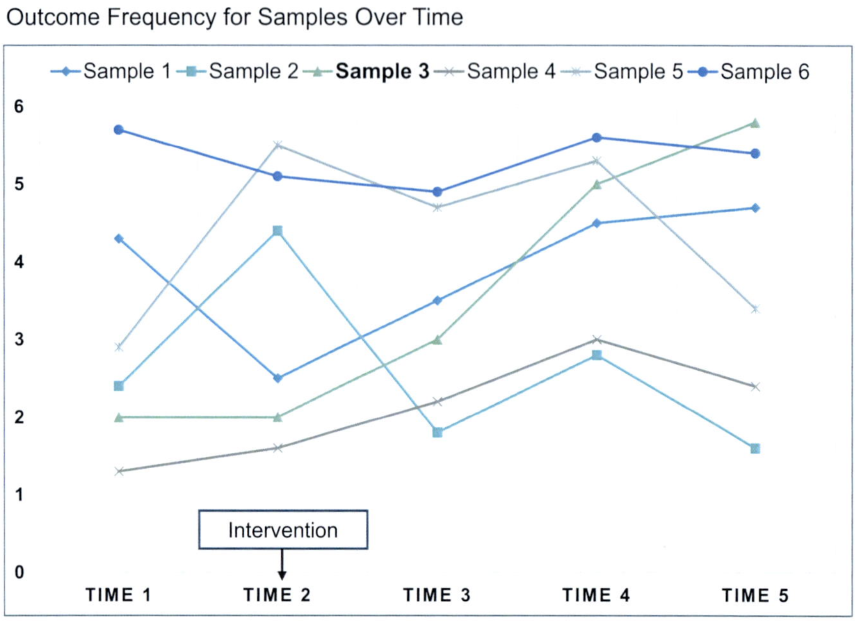

Fig. 11.1 Sufficient figure example one

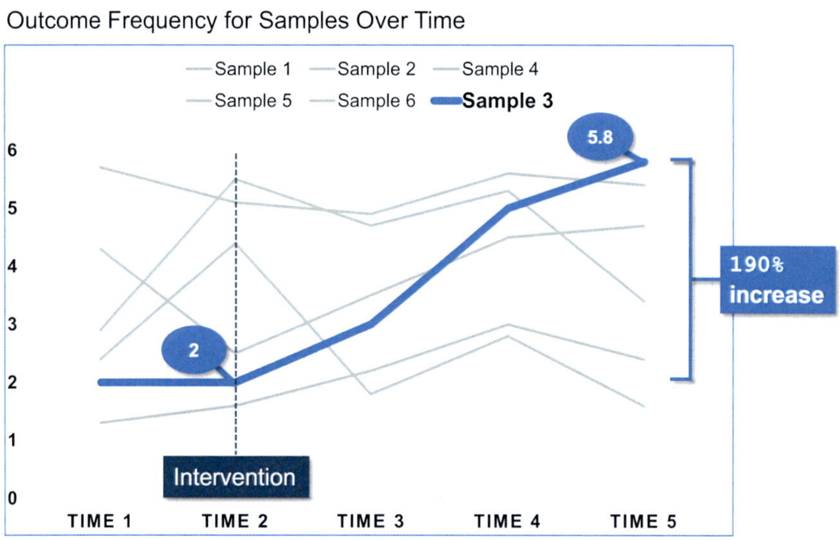

Fig. 11.2 Better figure example one

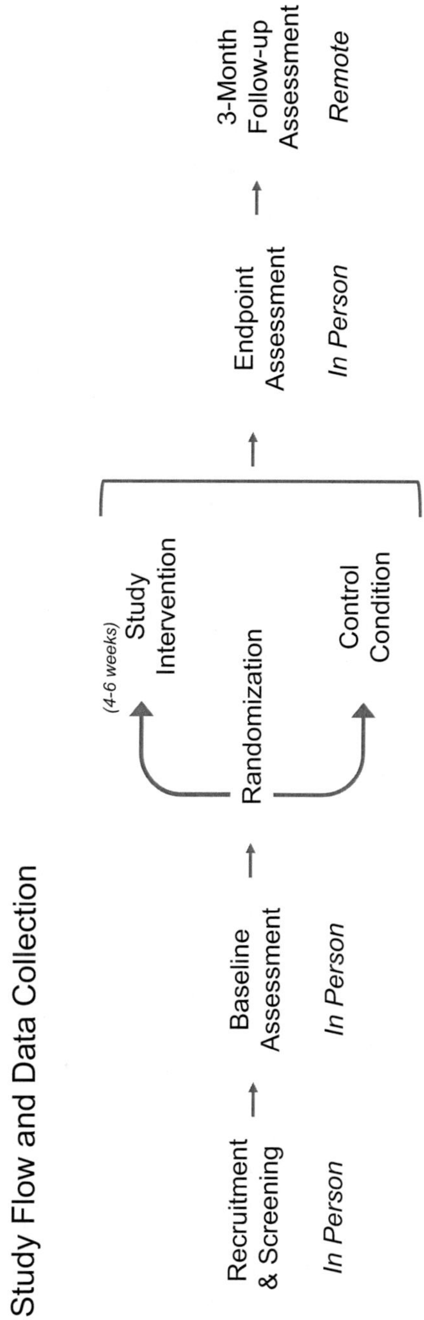

Fig. 11.3 Sufficient figure example two

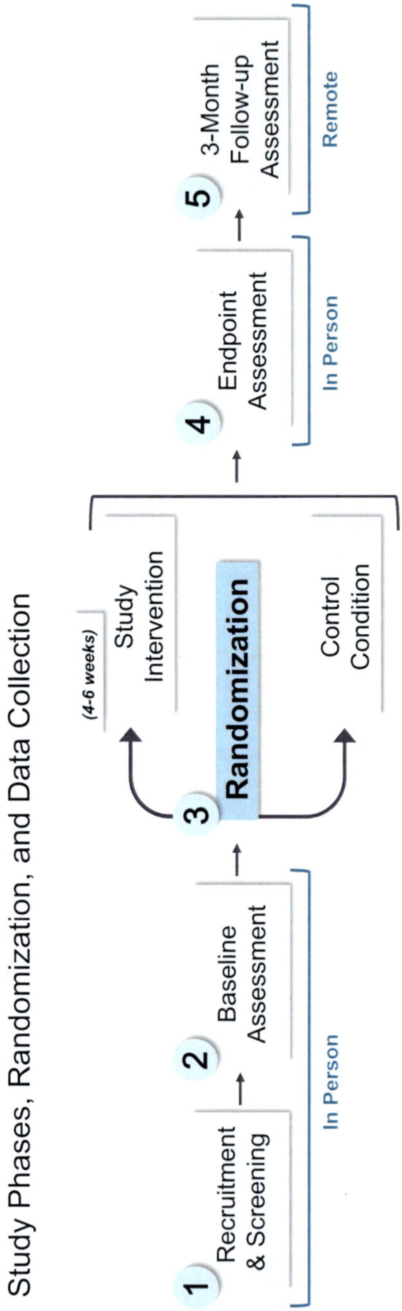

Fig. 11.4 Better figure example two

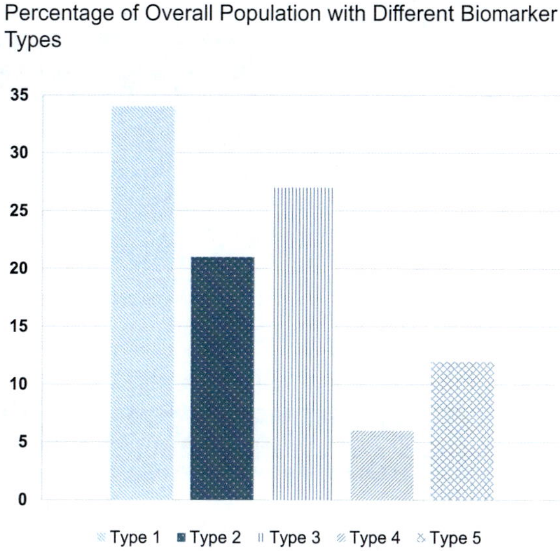

Fig. 11.5 Sufficient figure example three

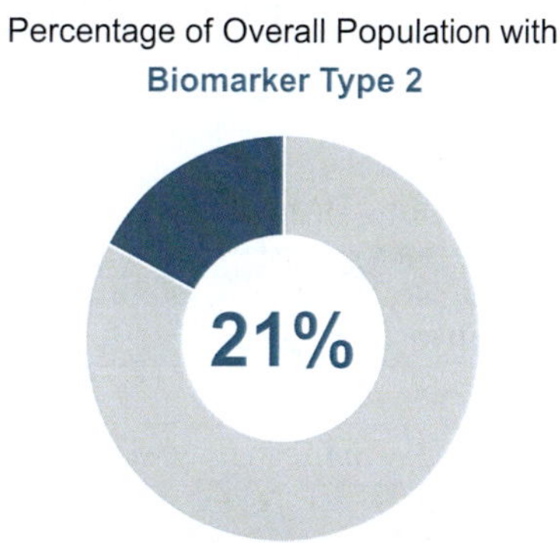

Fig. 11.6 Better figure example three

Comparison of Samples, with Significance

Sample Type	OR[a] (95% CI[b])	P-Value[c]
Type A	5.73 (1.39-17.69)	0.0030
Type B	4.18 (0.26-15.05)	0.0602
Type C	7.84 (2.58-19.06)	<0.0001
Type D	2.92 (-1.47-6.33)	0.1935
Type E	1.36 (-3.01-5.48)	0.2817

[a] OR = odds ratio; [b] CI = confidence interval; [c] univariate regression (Time 3 vs. Time 1 + Time 2)

Fig. 11.7 Sufficient table example one

Fig. 11.8 Better table example one, version one

Comparison of Samples, with Significance

Sample Type	Odds Ratio (95% Confidence Interval) & Significance[a]
Type A	**5.73 (1.39-17.69)***
Type B	4.18 (0.26-15.05)
Type C	**7.84 (2.58-19.06)****
Type D	2.92 (-1.47-6.33)
Type E	1.36 (-3.01-5.48)

[a] univariate regression (Time 3 vs. Time 1 + Time 2); * p<0.01; ** p<0.0001

Samples with Significant Results

Sample Type	Odds Ratio (95% Confidence Interval) & Significance[a]
Type A	**5.73 (1.39-17.69)***
Type C	**7.84 (2.58-19.06)****

[a] univariate regression (Time 3 vs. Time 1 + Time 2); * p<0.01; ** p<0.0001

Fig. 11.9 Better table example one, version two

Profits Before and After New Workflow

	Revenue*	Profits*
Two years prior	$639,000	$151,000
Prior year	$640,000	$152,000
Year 1 (shift to new workflow)	$495,000	$98,000
Year 2	$708,000	$216,000
Year 3	$923,000	$344,000
Year 4	$1,267,000	$503,000

*actual for prior years; predicted for years 1-4

Fig. 11.10 Sufficient table example two

Profit as Percent of Revenue Before and After New Workflow

	Revenue*	Profit*
Two years prior	$639,000	24%
Prior year	$640,000	24%
Year 1 ← **shift to new workflow**	$495,000	20%
Year 2	$708,000	**31%**
Year 3	$923,000	**37%**
Year 4	$1,267,000	**40%**

*actual for prior years; predicted for years 1-4

Fig. 11.11 Better table example two

References

Merriam-Webster. (2026). *Dictionary*. Retrieved January 31, 2026 from https://www.merriam-webster.com/dictionary/spin

National Cancer Institute. (n.d.) Retrieved September 4, 2023 from https://cancercontrol.cancer.gov/sites/default/files/2020-06/SGA_8704096.pdf (Ramaswamy, Megha, prinicipal investigator)

Chapter 12
Budget and Other Supporting Documents

12.1 Budgets

When I begin a proposal, I create two documents and work on them simultaneously: the overview that describes the specific aims and the budget. Why do this when many people save the budget until later? Because money drives what you can do. A rare funding organization supports an unlimited budget. Smaller grant mechanisms always have budget caps. This means that, despite what some people claim and what you may have been taught in school, you cannot let science completely drive how you write your aims and objectives. You *must* keep one eye on how much money you will have, because this, at least in part, defines the scope of your work.

Is this ideal? No. But it is realistic. Doing this up front avoids the pitfall of developing aims that do not match the budgetary constraints of the funding announcement. Imagine you are an early career biochemist and want to apply for a pilot funding mechanism, for which the maximum budget is $50,000 per year for two years. Up to now in your career, you only received a $5,000 intra-departmental grant. The pilot's budget thus seems like a small fortune.

As you determine your proposal's aims, you consider the budget. Your goal is to fund part of your salary and part of a lab technician's time. But you also hope to purchase small bench-scale equipment (a higher-quality centrifuge, calibrated pipettes, a reliable gel system, incubator, etc.) that would cost up to $5,000. You need reagents, preferably high-performance affinity resins, which you expect will run about $2,000. And you would like to support your future ability to do data analysis, graphing, and molecular-visualization and structure-viewing, which would mean investing over $2,000 in software. Finally, your colleagues warn you that core service fees at your university may tack as much as $10,000 per year onto your budget. Suddenly, $50,000 per year feels considerably less jaw-dropping.

Your early number crunching drives home how aims and budget interrelate and that items within a budget affect one another. If you stand firm on needing all equipment and software to do the aims, then you face a choice about where the rest of the

C. W. Hartmann, *Grant Writing Fundamentals Made Easy*,
https://doi.org/10.1007/978-3-032-35723-6_12

money goes. Do you fund less of your own salary and concentrate on supporting a lab technician? Will this change the quality of the work or the ability to gather the data that you want? If you fund more of yourself and less of a lab technician, will you have to perform more of the hands-on, day-to-day jobs? How will this affect whether you produce manuscripts and write other grants? These are questions and trade-offs better considered early.

Here is another example. Imagine you are an early career anthropologist interested in writing a mentored award for career development. The three-year award has a budget with enough money to cover your salary, but it only offers $30,000 per year for other expenses. You thought the budgeting would be easy and left it until close to the submission deadline. Your aims involve doing a large-scale quantitative survey and using those findings to inform many qualitative interviews. At least, that is how you wrote it. But as you look at quotes from vendors who administer surveys, you realize you cannot do as large a survey as you planned because you do not have the money to pay for it. You also hoped to support a research assistant to help you with interviews and data analysis, but you did not consider how much a research assistant would cost. You suddenly recognize you will have to do most of the interviews, data analysis, and write-ups yourself. This raises multiple issues, including the question of whether reviewers will believe you have time to do everything in your plan.

At the last minute, you change your aims. You reduce the survey's sample size, meaning that you must modify the methods section, arguing how the smaller survey provides meaningful information. You redo the power calculation and change the proposed analyses. You also have to justify a smaller number of interviews and explain how this number will result in important data. You thought you would have an easy submission. Instead, you struggle at the last minute, revisiting the literature and soliciting advice from colleagues.

As you can see from these examples, like it or not, budgets influence project execution. Developing them requires an investment of resources. So begin early to have time for adjustments and interplay between the science and the numbers.

12.2 Budget Justifications

Budget justifications assure funding organizations that every requested cost is reasonable, appropriate, and aligned with a proposal's aims and methods. Funding organizations usually provide instructions, so read and follow the requirements. Online or using AI, you can also find tips for how to construct justifications for various items, as well as successful examples. Even if you delegate the writing of this section to someone else, the final draft requires your review, because a mistake here can lead reviewers to question your proposal's adequacy.

Organize your justification as clearly as you construct the narrative sections of the proposal. (See Chap. 8, Sect. 8.3 and Chap. 11 for more on constructing these sections.) Budget justifications do not ordinarily have page limits, so use white space and headings to improve reviewers' cognitive ease. If the funding organization requires a form that enables text formatting, insert bullets or bold type when appropriate.

The decisive word for this section is "justification." Avoid simply describing items, assuming reviewers will know why you included them. Use this section as an *extension* of your main narrative. Succinctly and persuasively substantiate the need for each item, linking back to the aims or methods. When appropriate, tie things to the larger purpose and funding organization's priorities. Ensure a reader will understand not only *what* you want but *why* you need it. When doing this, be realistic. Ask for only as much as necessary, not more or less. Unreasonable requests (either too much or too little) can erode confidence in your project management abilities or the overall approach.

Before submission, match the items and numbers in the budget justification exactly to the budget. If you are lucky enough to have individuals helping you with a submission, request that they review the documents before finalization. Errors point to carelessness and lack of adequate oversight. Avoid giving reviewers the impression that you did not spend enough time on a document that undergirds your funding request.

12.3 Describing Personnel, Management Plans, and Environments

As with budget justifications, tips abound online on how to write personnel, management plan, and environment sections of a grant. But much less frequently discussed is how to use these to make a compelling case for your choice of team and working environment. Regardless of the way a funding organization wants this information presented, you have wiggle room.

Think of these sections as you would think about a resume. When you apply for a job, common advice is to customize your resume to the position. You can employ key terms from the job description, emphasize what the position requires and de-emphasize what it does not and endeavor to make yourself stand out, whether your resume is looked at by humans or AI. If nothing else, follow the 1–3-2/2-3-1 principle (see Chap. 7, Sect. 7.1). Help readers remember main points by putting them first and last. There are also other ways to customize.

12.3.1 Personnel

For describing personnel, many funding organizations in the US and elsewhere require the use of the electronic forms available through the US National Institutes of Health. Their "biosketch" form is frequently requested for individuals named in a proposal. It pulls information about publications from electronic records. But it also includes "personal statement" and "contributions to science" sections. You may have generic text for these sections that you recycle with each submission. A wiser approach involves tailoring these sections for yourself and your collaborators, aligning them with the content and goals of the application. For funding organizations that do not use a biosketch format, this is also true for any similar material.

The personal statement, in particular, offers extreme flexibility. Concentrate here on aspects of your training, skills, and career that are particularly relevant. Emphasize collaborations with other colleagues who are involved. Demonstrate that you are the right person for this work. Explain anything about your history that may puzzle reviewers (see Chap. 11, Sect. 11.6). Regardless of your discipline, this section enables you to tell a reviewer a convincing and memorable story. Start and end it with your most important points. And, if you are comfortable, try telling a tale that engages curiosity or emotions.

My own research centers on the quality and safety of care provided in nursing homes. For a grant about improving nursing home care for which I was principal investigator, here is how I started and ended the personal statement section of my biosketch. You may feel uncomfortable with such self-revelation. But, as you read, recognize my goal: to have a reviewer believe and remember why I am committed to this line of research.

> My interest in improving the quality of care in nursing homes extends back almost twenty years. The reason is personal. In 2005, my father had a massive hemorrhagic stroke from which he never recovered. He spent the last three years of his life in a nursing home. I chose his residence carefully, trying to ensure staff provided high-quality care in a person-centered environment, but when it mattered most, the home's culture failed him. In 2008, stomach flu raged through my father's building. When he was most ill, staff left him alone in his room, reclined in a chair, listening to Mozart. They honored his preferences as identified on his care plan: solitude and personalized music. But they did not simultaneously prioritize his safety. My father vomited. He could not reposition himself. He aspirated. Pneumonia followed. Two days later, he died.
>
> [Information pertaining to my credentials and their relevance to the grant came here.]
>
> Because of what happened to my father, I possess an unwavering, personal commitment to this proposal and a deep motivation to contribute to all areas of the proposed work.

Each application is unique. But think of a personal statement as more than a collection of facts. Think of it as an opportunity to relate a compelling story. This principle applies equally to bench science, social science, and humanities. Tie evidence you present to the proposal's main ideas, methods, trajectory of work, or team. Help reviewers remember and believe that you and your collaborators are the right people to undertake the project.

The other part of the biosketch that lends itself well to customization is the contributions to science section. In keeping with the 1-3-2/2-3-1 principle (see Chap. 7, Sect. 7.1), it should begin and end with the contributions most relevant to the *current* proposal. Do not recycle an order from a prior application if it does not fit. Edit text describing a contribution, linking each to an aspect of the current project. Change the publications you cite to highlight work with collaborators, familiarity with a methodology, or relevant, high-impact findings. Reviewers want to know what you have achieved and how that supports this submission.

12.3.2 Management Plan

Funding organizations have various requirements for how to present information about the proposal's team and resources. In general, instructions usually require a description of the team's structure and the roles individuals and groups will play in supporting a successful outcome. The space allotted for this varies. Ask colleagues for successful examples, preferably from proposals that were funded by the same organization. Before beginning to write, investigate how reviewers evaluate this section. What do the review criteria mention? Think about how best to follow the instructions and simultaneously address reviewers' needs. Sometimes this involves designing a table or an organizational chart. If that works, can you use color or shading to emphasize important aspects, making the graphic easy to understand quickly? (See Chap. 11, Sect. 11.7 for more on figures and tables.) Perhaps you only have room for a short paragraph. What pieces come first and last? Convince reviewers that your team will succeed.

12.3.3 Environment

Of all grant sections, this ranks among the most frequently recycled. Yes, many aspects of your environment will be similar across proposals because institutions remain constant. But what are reviewers truly looking for in this section?

Examine the review criteria again, pulling out pieces that directly or indirectly point to information to include. Ensure that what you describe matches what reviewers need to see to advocate for your project. Emphasize how each environment is aligned with and supports *this specific proposal.* If reviewers notice this section has been customized, they are more likely to read it in detail, meaning that during the review committee meeting they will remember more about why you are in the right situation to conduct the work.

No section of a grant is a "throwaway." Yes, some are more important than others. But each one contributes to the review. Give yourself time to modify every section according to the application's goals. Doing so improves the reviewer's experience. And it heightens the chance of creating a positive impression of not only your attention to detail but also of your ability to manage large tasks.

Chapter 13
Resubmission

This chapter is about how to navigate the process of resubmission within the context of cognitive ease. Not long ago, I sat on a multiday grant review panel. We met over Zoom, with time zones spanning the US. For some of us, the meeting began in the middle of the night, for others mid-morning. Each day, our group discussed about ten applications, including numerous reapplications. Each proposal had three assigned reviewers. For the reapplications, these were frequently the same people who had been assigned to the proposal's prior submission. But sometimes a few or all were different.

The reapplication package included the critique statement from the previous review. This comprised the summary points from the discussion of the full committee, if applicable, and the comments of each previously assigned reviewer. During the panel discussion, my fellow reviewers and I *always* mentioned these prior critiques.

Imagine you were on the panel. You too might say, "This application was very responsive to the prior review." Your brow might wrinkle if you encountered an applicant who pushed back on the previous reviewers' opinions and declined to make a change. You might observe, "A previous reviewer already noted this issue, but I saw no improvement in the current application." Even over Zoom, you would notice that calm voices sometimes gave way to edgy tones and curt impatience when discussing an unresponsive proposal.

Reviewers are ethical and well-intentioned. They comment on proposals because they believe in the process of peer-review. They are also human. They appreciate feeling valued, especially when they spend hours thinking critically about whether arguments are sound. Each reapplication is judged on its own merits, but partly within the context of how well it acknowledges what reviewers said before.

My own emotional reaction to a reapplication begins when I read the synopsis of revisions made in response to the prior review. Does that document promote cognitive ease or is it crammed with text I find difficult to follow? Do new objectives and outcomes clearly relate to the funding organization's *current* priorities? How often does the applicant *resist* reviewers' suggestions without convincing me of the

C. W. Hartmann, *Grant Writing Fundamentals Made Easy*,
https://doi.org/10.1007/978-3-032-35723-6_13

validity of their stance? Do I feel an undertone of, "I [the applicant] was right the first time, and you [the reviewer] should accept that," creating a figurative tug of war?

Understandably, an applicant may first react negatively upon receiving an opportunity to resubmit. Among other things, resubmission means no immediate funding, additional work, a delay in any plans tied to the original proposal, and another unknown outcome at the end of the process. Initially, applicants can feel disgruntled, discouraged, or even angry. Yet a chance for resubmission means the door is still open. In my experience, the best attitude when crafting a resubmission is gratitude. That feeling then permeates the modifications and any description of those. Reviewers notice the tone. And one of the criteria by which resubmissions are often judged is responsiveness to prior critiques.

13.1 Deciding How to Respond

I suggest beginning the revision process by constructing a table, as described in more detail below. This starts with a simple cut and paste exercise to transfer each negative comment into a cell. Deciding how to *respond* to those comments is a complex art, with no single correct answer. The following can help you make decisions.

Read between the lines. If you are stumped by reviewers' thoughts, reach out to seasoned colleagues and those who sit on grant review panels. Ask them specific questions such as, "What do you think the reviewer meant by XYZ? Is there a hidden message I might be missing?" or, "In light of the summary comments (or the score), what would you do if you received this comment from Reviewer 1 and that comment from Reviewer 2?" You can also ask AI, but that entails risks, not the least of which has to do with AI's inability to take larger contexts into account, including those surrounding the application itself, the state of the science, and the priorities of the funding organization. AI also tends to tell you what it thinks you want to hear, making it less useful in this situation. (For more on using AI in grant writing, see Chap. 1, Sect. 1.3.) Preferably, rely on people to help you find a way through the fog. Gather colleagues or your proposal team for a quick meeting or email exchange, sharing your response table and questions. Getting other brains involved often results in clarity or a path forward.

Only fix what is broken. With fresh eyes, you may see holes in your application no reviewer noticed. You may want to make small improvements, do things differently, or even enact larger changes than called for by the prior critiques. If you do this, avoid raising new issues or red flags. What seems to you like an improvement may disorient reviewers or cause them to think, "If the first revision had this error, maybe there are others I didn't notice." Fix cosmetic or minor flaws without drawing attention to them. But unless solving a larger one is necessary because it is fatal or related to another change you make in response to the critiques, a general rule of thumb is to respond comprehensively, thoughtfully, and appreciatively to the prior review and not much beyond it.

Assess the need for additional data. Reviewers are often instructed not to tell you how to fix the issues they bring up. You may have to decide whether their comments indicate the need for a better use of existing data or whether performing further preliminary work to collect new data would bolster your case in the resubmission. And as Chip and Dan Heath mention in their book *Switch: How to Change Things When Change is Hard* (2010), what appears to be resistance may also be a lack of clarity. In other words, reviewers may dispute your ideas simply because your original descriptions were not clear. You might not need any additional data at all, just a better explanation of the data you do have. If you speak with an official from the funding organization, you can ask about this. You can also discuss this with your colleagues and team.

Talk with someone from the funding organization. If you understand the main themes within the comments and realize you have specific questions, contact the person in charge of the review process. They cannot write the revision for you, divulge information about reviewers or the content of the review panel meeting, or hold your hand multiple times. But they may be able to give an overall sense of reviewers' enthusiasm for the ideas and answer general questions about positioning a revision in light of current funding organization priorities. Avoid putting them on the spot or pushing them if they are hesitant to respond. But do feel empowered to contact them unless this is specifically forbidden by a particular organization. This type of discussion is usually a normal part of the reapplication process.

Assess the need for more time. Sometimes you choose to avoid resubmitting immediately and instead resubmit in a later review cycle. You may reach that decision easily because it is indicated by your score, the magnitude of the changes necessitated, or the need for more data or preliminary work. But at times the decision to delay creeps up on you gradually. Sometimes writers pull back from submitting as late as a few days before the deadline (see Chap. 5, Sect. 5.4). If your proposal is not the best you can make it, consider waiting.

The reviewers are always right. As noted above, your attitude toward the revision matters. Reviewers smell anger and resentment a mile away. If you decide you must disagree, employ the 1–3-2/2-3-1 principle (see Chap. 7, Sect. 7.1) and do it in the middle. Then, revisit your answer and try not to push back at all.

Start early. This is not news by now, but to write a strong reapplication, you must begin a revision early, even as soon as the day you get the comments from the prior submission. (See Chap. 3, Sect. 3.3 for more on the importance of starting early.)

13.2 How to Construct a Revisions Table

A table of comments and responses guides changes you make. It also serves as the starting point for any response document you may need to submit with your reapplication.

One format is pictured in Table 13.1. (I included alphabetic letters in column headings only for ease of explanation; they do not belong in an actual table.) In this table, the numbering system in column A helps reference comments and responses for yourself if some content repeats. Column B is used later for the organization of rows by themes, such as "significance of the work," "feasibility," or "methodological concerns." Column C exists because a proposal often receives comments from more than one reviewer and frequently also receives a summary statement about the review process. Columns D and E are for the reviewer critiques and your responses to them.

To begin, highlight the critique document. I recommend doing this electronically. Read the entire document, highlighting *every negative* statement. You can also ask AI to do this for you, but check its work if you do. Split issues apart. If, for example, the summary document indicates multiple problems with the methods, highlight each problem individually. After going through the entire document, read it again, looking for negative things you (or AI) missed.

End this experience on a positive note. Using a different color or method, highlight any positive statements, particularly searching for ones to tone down any negativity. If Reviewer 2 had doubts about your novel data collection tool but Reviewer 1 praised your innovation and thought the tool would work, highlight Reviewer 1's points. You may use this in your response.

Next, populate columns C and D with information from the critique document, beginning with any summary of the review process you received. Leave columns A and B blank for now. Include all negative or critical comments verbatim. This means using the exact text from the review with as much surrounding text as you need to make the comment comprehensible without looking back at the original document. Include positive comments if, as noted above, you think they bolster your responses. Be thorough in quoting the critiques.

For some funding organizations, the summary of the review process is much more important than individual reviewers' comments because the summary captures the discussion among the panel members, while the individual critiques were written before the panel met. The table you construct may need only the summary document comments, or it may need those plus individual reviewers' thoughts. If you only received reviewer comments, it will include only those. If you are unsure of the weight to give to summary versus individual comments, ask successful, experienced colleagues or a program official at the funding organization.

The number of rows depends, of course, on the number of critiques. Avoid being daunted by the number or by redundancy, which will be sorted out later. At this stage, accurate cutting and pasting is the goal. Once you fill in all possible information, the table becomes the primary document from which you construct your response.

The next step is to ensure that each row contains only one issue. A comment may combine two points, where each requires a different response. A critique may

Table 13.1 Example 1

A. Point #	B. Theme	C. Who said it	D. Verbatim critique	E. Response
–	–	–	–	–
–	–	–	–	–

indicate, "Major concerns regarding the feasibility of the intervention and the power calculation." Initially, you might copy this into one row because a reviewer wrote it as one sentence. But upon rereading, you note that a response to "duration of the intervention" would be different from that for "the power calculation." In this case, you would separate the comments into two different rows.

Work on column B next. There are themes hidden within your table. Your job is to find them, step by step.

First, move all similar statements next to each other by cutting and pasting rows so that related, analogous, or repetitive comments are above and below each other. (Now you understand why you did not number the comments in column A yet.) Because you have exact quotes and have a column for who said what, the table will always identify the essential information, no matter how much you reorganize.

Second, think about how those grouped ideas hang together. What is the common theme that prompted you to move them near one another? Create a merged row spanning all columns that identifies each theme. When doing this, pause to consider whether you label a theme based on exactly what the reviewers said or whether you are needlessly or incorrectly extrapolating.

The process you do here is similar to a process in qualitative research called "coding," where an interview is analyzed for information that is summarized into snippets or "codes." When coding the content of an interview, a researcher often wants to stay as close to the words of the interviewee as possible and not make their own interpretations. For example, imagine coding an interviewee comment such as, "My situation was unique. There were so many things that happened only to me and not to anybody else." A code that sticks to the interviewee's words and meaning might be "unique situation." Codes that interpret or extrapolate might be "feels alone" or "self-centered."

When writing your themes about reviewer comments, stick to what was said, not what you *think* might lie far behind the words. Do not jump to hypothesizing. Make your themes easy for the next reviewers to follow. They may not be the same people.

Often, initial themes are evident. Be open to others. Note that comments may fall under more than one theme; it is fine to duplicate a row, placing it in more than one place. Some comments might need further splitting because they contain multiple issues that do not fit within only one theme. And some may not fit within any theme. You can group these into an "Other comments" theme or divide them into "Other major" and "Other minor" themes. It is also fine to have critiques that stand alone. The goal is to aggregate as much as logically possible. When in doubt about what falls under which theme, recruit colleagues or AI to help assess the points. Often writers find it necessary to tweak themes as they go. You may merge, subdivide, edit, or create subthemes that fall under a larger one (for example, you may have a larger theme of "Data Collection Issues" and have subthemes of "Survey Distribution," "Interviewee recruitment," and "Interviewer Training"). It might take several iterations to organize the content.

The last step is to order the themes. Move the most important to the top. Judge importance by how important *reviewers* thought a theme was and how much relative weight a funding organization places on the summary statement, if you received one. If critiques from a summary statement have precedence, these belong at the beginning. If comments from Reviewers 2 and 3 restate or expand on what is covered in a summary comment, move the reviewer comments below the summary comment point. These may become subthemes or be merged into the summary comment theme. Keep the least important things until the end. (This is one time to *ignore* the 1–3-2 / 2-3-1 principle of placing the most important things first and last (see Chap. 7, Sect. 7.1 for more on this principle)).

Realize that we all tend to gravitate either to lumping or splitting. This means that some of us prefer fewer themes and lump loosely related topics together. Others like ideas to remain separate and end up splitting topics into many themes. Understand your own preferences and then decide how many themes, presented in what order, will be easiest for *reviewers* to understand. Keep the curse of knowledge (see Chap. 7, Sect. 7.2) in mind as you do this. Have a colleague inspect the themes to see whether the table's content and order make sense.

After you finalize themes and their order, fill in column A. Table 13.2 presents an abbreviated version of a table with themes. I inserted an extra row above each theme to identify and separate them.

13.3 Your Responses in the Table

For a revision, the most important column is E, where you indicate how you respond. Several simple principles can improve how you craft the responses. Each requires imagining yourself in the position of a reviewer.

13.3.1 Principle 1: Use the Same Words

Avoid making reviewers hunt for information in the revised application and in any response document. You may not have a lot of space. And yet it is vital that reviewers identify words and phrases from the prior critiques in what you write because that will help them believe you understood the comments and responded.

Use key words that reviewers and the summary statement used. If the previous review stated, "Issues related to sampling raise questions of generalizability," use some of this phrasing. Indicate how you changed your "sampling" methods, leading to increased "generalizability." If they said, "It's unclear how the proposed final product would be implemented in practice," you might start by writing that you "clarified" the viability of "implementation in practice" by [fill in the methods]. You get the idea.

You may struggle with this principle because someone once taught you that repetition is a sign of laziness or bad writing. But in writing responses to critiques, you have only one goal: increase the ease with which reviewers find information, believe your arguments, and can advocate for your application. Using their exact words and

Table 13.2 Example 2

A. Point #	B. Theme	C. Who said it	D. Verbatim critique	E. Response
Significance				
1	Significance	Key summary point	Not clear that application of the principal investigator's prior study is appropriate for this population.	
2	Significance	Reviewer 1	[it] is not clear that replication is appropriate for this setting.	
Feasibility				
3	Feasibility	Key summary point	Major concerns about the approach (e.g.,… underreporting of the primary outcome).	
4	Feasibility	Reviewer 3	Would be helpful to have the annual rates for the primary outcome variable.	
5	Feasibility	Reviewer 3	Impact of the study is not convincing, as it is unclear whether the impact of intervention on the primary outcome can be assessed.	
Power calculation				
6		Key summary point	Major concerns about the approach (e.g.,… weak justification for power calculation).	
7	Power calculation	Reviewer 2	Clarifying the assumptions behind the power calculation would be helpful.	
Intervention sustainment				
8	Intervention sustainment	Key summary point	Study would be strengthened with a methodology for a longer follow-up.	

(continued)

Table 13.2 (continued)

A. Point #	B. Theme	C. Who said it	D. Verbatim critique	E. Response
9	Intervention sustainment	Reviewer 2	It would be useful to do a longer-term assessment of sustainment in wave 1 sites. Three to six months is not actually long enough in terms of sustainability of the intervention.	
10	Intervention sustainment	Reviewer 3	As this is a 4-year project, I would rather see fewer sites with longer follow-up	
Data collection issues				
11	Data collection	Key summary point	Major concerns about the …methods section	
Data collection tools—Qualitative				
12	Data collection tools—Qualitative	Reviewer 2	It would be nice to see something from this project that could increase the organization's capacity to do these kinds of partnerships	
13	Data collection—Qualitative	Reviewer 2	What if the site does not use the intervention? Are those interview questions skipped?	
Data collection tools—Quantitative				

(continued)

Table 13.2 (continued)

A. Point #	B. Theme	C. Who said it	D. Verbatim critique	E. Response
14	Data collection—Quantitative	Reviewer 1	There is little information about the instrument "site-level integration rating template" (appendix 6). This seems an important instrument but there is no reliability or validity information and it is not clear how it will be used in the overall evaluation.	
15		Reviewer 1	Not doing a relational coordination survey at the height of the implementation seems like a missed opportunity to assess the conceptual model.	
Timing issues				
16	Timing issues	Reviewer 1	It looks like all intervention tailoring will happen before any intervention starts. This may be unrealistic.	
17	Timing issues	Reviewer 2	The intervention implementation is currently slated to start year 2, quarter 2. This means there is a lot of qualitative data collection at the back end, and I wonder if 4 years is sufficient.	

phrases helps do this, whether in a response document or the revised proposal. We all like people who listen to our advice.

13.3.2 Principle 2: Be Unequivocal

A successful response leaves the impression that all revisions are well grounded. Of course, when appropriate, indicate that you considered other options. Then finish your arguments with an explanation of why what you decided is best. To do this, avoid clauses and phrases that imply equivocation or conditions. Sentences that begin with words such as "although," "while," "despite," "even though," and "notwithstanding" imply contrast and bury the lede.

13.3.3 Principle 3: Do Not Push Back

Remember that reviewer criticism may indicate a lack of clarity in your initial submission. Avoid berating or blaming people for not noticing something that was already spelled out in the prior application. Take a close look at where you believe you explained it and what they critiqued. Find a way to clarify the issue. Perhaps the information was in the middle of a paragraph or buried within a section. Revise to draw reviewers' attention to it. (Section 13.7.2 shows a response that addresses something already described in a prior submission.)

Reviewers comment on an application because they think it can improve. Tamp down any impulse to refute, ignore, or disparage a reviewer's position. Address everything they bring up (or at least the major points), and do it respectfully. If a reviewer is off base or wrong, you can still find ways to address the issue without sounding arrogant or dismissive.

In a grant, my team and I once proposed using cognitive interviews to refine a draft survey. Cognitive interviewing, despite the name, is *not* a traditional qualitative data collection technique. It does not involve traditional interviewing. It is an established method in survey development that, in our case, required having individuals think aloud as they answered the draft survey.

But one of the reviewers was a qualitative researcher and saw the word "interview" and equated it with qualitative research. They called into question our sample size, data collection methods, and analysis. This was a misunderstanding on their part. But we chose to own it as a failure in communication on our part. In response to reviews and in the revised application, we said that we would conduct "think aloud exercises" and removed all instances of the word "interview." We provided examples of how think aloud exercises work and cited sources that substantiated our data collection and analysis choices, explaining why we rejected alternative methods and how ours were the most viable, established, and rigorous. We avoided explicitly indicating we had changed our methods, because we had not. But we did use wording that someone could read as a change if they wanted to. For example, "In this application we will use think aloud exercises…" The reviewer accepted this. The proposal was funded.

Exercise: Rephrase for Authoritativeness

Rephrase the following. Use multiple sentences if needed. Have each sentence focus on only one point.

- Although the XYZ method is more common in our field, we chose to employ ABC.
- While our population of interest has a higher incidence of several pressing health concerns, diabetes represents a critical one to study for many reasons that we describe below.
- Despite the difficulties inherent in our approach, we believe it is best and will ensure success.

In many cases, you can eliminate the beginning of such sentences. State your position or conclusion first, before contrasting it with another. This will ensure that reviewers are more likely to remember what you plan to do rather than what you do not. Here are the above examples, rewritten.

- We will employ the ABC method because it has distinct advantages over more common methods, such as XYZ. [Continue with reasons supporting your position, such as, "Recent studies show the ABC method is stronger at detecting change. It is also simpler to use, resulting in less error."]
- Diabetes is a critical health concern for our population of interest. [After this, list the reasons it is important to study, perhaps also adding its relationship to other health concerns this population has.]
- We chose our approach because [demonstrate why this is a wise choice, including facts about what this approach has enabled in similar situations]. The following methods will ensure that we are able to overcome any difficulties. [List each potential difficulty and the methods by which you will anticipate and overcome it. This does not need to be excruciatingly detailed; give reviewers enough information to believe you.] [End with a positive statement, such as, "Coupling our proven approach with strong methods will ensue the success of our study."]

13.4 Finalizing Your Responses

The overarching goal of a revision is to respond to both the letter *and spirit* of every important comment and create a new proposal that exceeds the cognitive ease of the prior submission. The process of deciding what needs to change and how to present new information is not a science but an art. There are many possible variations, each valuable to the extent that it answers a concern and is easy for the next reviewers to understand and accept.

At this stage in the revision process, you are no longer thinking only of your table. You are also involved in an iterative process of revising your application. Changes in the proposal inform the content of the responses in the table and vice versa. Responses also frequently require adding text to the application, even though the original space limitations usually remain in place. (See Chap. 14 for tips on cutting text.)

Relying on the organized information in the table, craft responses in column E. As you do this, you may, for example, address point number three (the point numbers are in column A) and realize that the same content reappears in point number seven. If so, jot a note in number seven that says, "See response to #3." But be careful. Sometimes, there are subtle differences that must be addressed separately.

After drafting initial responses, ask colleagues or AI (if allowable) to edit them. If you have a firm understanding of the comments and themes but cannot solve a specific issue, you might email a person at the funding organization.

13.4.1 Tips for Drafting Responses in the Table

- Begin with a broad pass at the entire table.
- Use bullets to outline your initial strategy within a theme. Worry less about wording. Use phrases and short sentences to describe a response within or across comments. After solidifying a main strategy across a theme, dive in more deeply.
- Color-code responses by how easy they are to address. Use, for example, one color for easy-to-address ones, another for those you find more difficult, and yet a different one for those where you need outside help. Change the colors once you and your colleagues are satisfied with the answer.
- Avoid immediately making substantial changes to the proposal's text. Wait until the table response is fleshed out. When you do make changes in the text, use track changes or another mechanism to highlight what you do. This enables you to easily identify modifications to reference later if you need.
- Note what comments likely drove the score. These are often ones that relate to areas where multiple reviewers agree and/or where the critique is strong and large. Move those to the top of each theme. Your answer must be visible quickly.
- Note where reviewers disagree and think carefully about how to address that. If you need to write a response document to describe your changes, you can sometimes lean on positive reviewer comments. If a few reviewers liked a method but one reviewer had a problem with it, you may be able to weave in some assistance, such as, "The ABC method, as pointed out by Reviewers 2 and 3, supports our primary goal of XYZ. We thus keep the overall method and, as suggested by Reviewer 1, modify it by…".

13.5 Creating a Response Document

If the resubmission calls for writing a formal response document that reacts to the prior review and describes the changes you made and why, build it around the themes and responses in the table. Find guidelines for this document applicable to the specific funding organization. Also ask successful colleagues for examples and look online to obtain others. Below are tips for how to draft your version.

Start with headings. Use your table to draft headings for the themes. Keep page limits in mind. Some organizations allow only one paragraph or page, while others allow more. What you say depends, in part, on how much room you have. Choose your headings accordingly.

Begin with an overview. Even if instructions limit word or page counts, begin with a sentence that orients reviewers to what you do in the remainder of the document. If you have more space, you might highlight a few positive comments, summarize critical revisions, touch on the major themes, or indicate how you will indicate locations in the main grant text that have changes.

Prioritize score-driving themes to which you have strong revisions. Respond first to the largest issues. Order these by how robust you believe your revisions are. For example, imagine you identify three major themes and feel confident about the way you address two of these. List these two first, even if reviewers or the summary document noted them later.

Sandwich smaller critical comments between less critical ones and your weakest responses between stronger ones. Here is an example of how you might phrase something. "Reviewer 2's critique was helpful. We considered X, Y, and Z as possible solutions. X and Y do not work in the case of this proposal because [list reasons]. We therefore will use Z, as it represents a rigorous and feasible method aligned with study goals that will ensure success by [include details of Z and how it will work]."

To the extent space allows, ensure all points are covered and all reviewers are included. If the document focuses on more than just the summary of the review meeting, acknowledge all contributors in the response. Sometimes, one or two reviewers drive most of the content. If you have space, also include input from the others, even if it means inserting a lesser critique or a positive comment. Nobody likes to feel ignored.

Think about layout. Recall the importance of cognitive ease. (See Chap. 1, Sect. 1.1 for more on cognitive ease.) Use direct quotes from critiques, indicated with quotation marks or italics, as much as possible, shortening them with ellipses when needed. This helps reviewers match their comments with your responses. For the same reason, if you paraphrase what reviewers said, still select some words reviewers used and insert them with quotation marks. Value white space. If you have room, generate subthemes to organize information. Consider using bullets or numbered lists. The more easily reviewers can find and understand your points, the better.

The end of this chapter includes abridged versions of two successful response documents.

13.6 Evaluating How You Feel

Emotional reactions, if unacknowledged, can hamper a successful revision. Every proposal writer understands that an opportunity to resubmit means they are one step closer to funding, a cause for celebration. But reading reviewer comments, particularly harsh ones, can engender negative feelings. This is normal.

Do what you need to do: grieve, rant, malign. Write nasty emails that you delete later. Call friends for support. Take a run. Let the emotions rise to the surface. Then, accept them and wait until they recede.

Avoid reading unwarranted criticism into reviewers' statements. What feels like reproach may simply be a usual type of wording that review committees use. If this was the first grant you ever submitted, and you think the critiques are uncommonly severe, step back for a reality check. Ask colleagues to share their grants' reviewer critiques. As you read those, assess whether your critiques are indeed tough or whether others' critiques have a similar tone or general content.

Also consider how you approach grant writing generally and a revision specifically. Do you have approach goals or avoidance goals? (Elliot, 2006) In other words, do you think, "I want to avoid another poor score" or "I don't want to make any mistakes in the revision" (avoidance goals)? Or do you think, "I want to use the reviewers' comments to make the proposal substantially better" or "I want to increase the likelihood that reviewers become enthusiastic about the project" (approach goals)? Being aware of your orientation helps you understand how you proceed with the revision process. (See Chap. 1, Sect. 1.1 for more on the avoidance-approach motivation framework.)

Imagine that one theme in your critiques is lack of convincing detail in the recruitment strategy. An avoidance orientation might mean you do not want reviewers to criticize recruitment again. This may lead to plugging holes, adding citations, and proving that every point that reviewers noted was addressed. This may attend to the issues but may also lack coherence within the overall design or sound defensive. An approach orientation, on the other hand, may lead to your trying to convince reviewers that the revised design is rigorous. This might lead to your crafting a compelling recruitment narrative, integrating it better into the overall design, making strengths more visible, and improving clarity and persuasiveness through added detail. One way to distinguish avoidance and approach in this example is to think of the former as removing weaknesses and the latter as increasing enthusiasm. These differences are subtle but may influence how reviewers react to a response.

Once you have done all this, put yourself into a reviewer's shoes by pretending you are a reviewer who reviewed a grant and participated in a grant review meeting. Envision the critique you wrote for that grant as though it were a special dinner you, the reviewer, cooked for the applicant. For that dinner, you thought about the menu ahead of time (read the reviewer instructions), bought all the ingredients (read the proposal), chopped and cooked everything (decided on and wrote up your comments), and presented the dishes in the most beautiful way you could (thoughtfully discussed the proposal during the grant review meeting).

Then, imagine that a dinner guest (the applicant) sits down and picks your meal apart, telling you what you did wrong. No appreciation, only complaints about the results of your hard work. How do you, as the cook (reviewer), feel?

And reviewers are not ordinary cooks. They are celebrity chefs chosen for their expertise and knowledge. They perform their work by special invitation. They hold the power to grade a dinner guest's behavior and decide whether the guest stays in the dining room or goes home.

So as the applicant, praise the cook's meal, even if you do not enjoy eating it. In the end, you may learn more from it than you thought. Most of all, remember the meal was prepared just for you and appreciate all the effort that went into that process.

13.7 Example Response Documents

Below are two abridged responses to critiques my teams received from initial submissions of different grants. We included them, as required, with the resubmissions. The responses both quote extensively from the summary we received about the panels' discussions. If our grants had not been discussed by a panel, the responses would have quoted only individual reviewers. Both grants were funded on resubmission. See what you think.

13.7.1 Example Response Document One

The first example is an abridged version of a response document submitted to the US National Institute on Aging. The quotes are from the summary critique that synthesized the content of the review groups' discussions. The response refers to reviewer comments when they align with themes from the summary. This document was limited to one page. Italics indicate the issues raised. Our responses follow.

1. *"The responsibilities of each member of the investigative [team] are challenging to delineate."*

   (a) Dr. X will join Dr. Y as a principal investigator via the multiple-principal investigator mechanism, and both will increase their percent effort. Dr. X, an implementation science expert, will assume a greater role in study oversight and management. This enables Dr. Y (as per Reviewers 1 & 2) to participate more closely and substantively in the nursing home field work, directly overseeing the creation of intervention material development and intervention delivery. Drs. X and Y have complementary expertise and have a successful multiple-principal investigator history [grant numbers included here]. We outline the delineation of roles in the multiple-principal investigator plan...

2. *"There's insufficient attention to power calculations and various parameters are not justified [also noted by Reviewer 2]. It's unclear whether the calculations are realistic or not, for this specific study and targeted population."*

   Our estimates of intervention effect size, eligible individuals per nursing home, and the likely intra-cluster correlation are realistic and evidence-based, taken from the work of the proposal's investigators and from the effects documented by other teams, as per the peer-reviewed dementia literature (research plan sect. E8). We calculate our power and sample size estimates using established procedures, now described in greater detail in sect. H2. We propose a stepped wedge design with standardized pre- and post-implementation data collection periods for each step to ensure the feasibility of data collection while capitalizing on the stepped wedge design's positive impact on statistical power…
3. *"The analysis plan does not discuss whether severity of dementia will be studied to identify its effect on effectiveness of the intervention."*

   We agree severity of dementia could be an important moderator and now include severity of dementia in the analysis as a moderator to examine whether the effects are different in various populations...

13.7.2 Example Response Document Two

The following example is from a response document for a submission to the US Department of Veterans Affairs (called "VA" in the document). The application was about implementing the "LOCK program" to improve nursing home care quality. This program rests on the foundation of frontline staff huddling (brief stand-up meetings) to build effective teamwork. The document is organized by theme, with the first themes coming from the summary critique written after the review group met. We also indicate where individual reviewers mentioned similar issues. Note that the response starts by addressing an issue that arose late in the summary critique. We moved it to the beginning of the response document because this was a critical issue to which we had a strong reply. The second issue addressed in the response document has to do with something that was already in the prior proposal. We wanted to clarify this as soon as possible. This document had a three-page limit. Again, italics indicate issues raised.

> We appreciate the thoughtful feedback on our first submission and are gratified by the consistent sense across critiques regarding strengths of the proposal as reflected in Summary points 1–3, including that the conceptual framework and study design are appropriate. We embraced the critiques' guidance and made changes to enhance the approach, site selection, innovation, and follow-up, along with responding to other points from individual reviewers. Below, we detail our responses to key themes and specific issues from each critique, also indicating where revisions are in the research plan.
>
> *Is "application of the principal investigator's prior study appropriate for...State Veterans Homes"? (Summary point 6; Reviewers 1 & 2).*
>
> As Reviewer 1 noted, a major impact of this research is "advanc[ing] the science on how…to intervene in a clinical setting that does not have a system-wide quality and safety program."

We nevertheless understand the reviewers' concerns about the extent of the variation in State Veterans Homes and the implicit worry about implementing our LOCK program intervention in sites that do not have a foundation for quality improvement. Unlike VA nursing homes, individual State Veterans Homes lack connection to hospital-level quality improvement support and have lacked a national quality improvement infrastructure. Yet this environment is exactly the one to which this proposal is geared. Our team has successfully implemented the LOCK program in VA's lowest performing nursing homes, which are arguably more like State Veterans Homes. Our implementation of the LOCK program principles has also improved care in many non-VA community nursing homes classified as "special focus" by the Centers for Medicare and Medicaid Services, i.e., homes with a history of serious, intransigent quality issues.

This is possible because the LOCK program *itself* is composed of fundamental quality improvement structures and processes and helps each nursing home create its own quality improvement system. It thereby avoids reliance on preexisting national or even strong local quality improvement infrastructures. Instead, the program builds culture from the bottom up through blended facilitation (researcher facilitators working with the site-based leadership team). The key ingredient at the site level is stable and engaged site-level leadership, which we incorporate into our site selection (sect. F.2.a.).

The revised proposal now does the following in response to reviewer comments.

1. Acknowledges the likely variation in State Veteran Home familiarity with and support for quality improvement (A.1.)
2. Delineates recent VA policies that are beginning to build a new, national State Veteran Home quality improvement infrastructure (A.2.). These policy changes will slowly grow a national State Veteran Home quality improvement infrastructure within which this grant proposal will operate but upon which this proposal avoids dependence due to the LOCK program's ability to create its own structures and processes at the site level.
3. …

   "Concerns about....annual fall rates...under reporting of falls...unclear explanation of how annual fall rates were used for the power calculation...weak justification for power calculation" (Summary point 4; Reviewers 2 & 3).

   We clarified throughout the application that our primary outcome has always been the rate of "fall during episode of care" (called "any fall") and eliminated early comparisons to "fall with major injury" that caused confusion. Any fall is the percent of State Veterans Home residents experiencing at least one fall of any type in the quarter. The new Table 1 indicates rates of any fall per quarter in State Veterans Homes, averaged across four quarters: on average, approximately 55% of residents in State Veterans Homes experienced at least one fall per quarter. Reviewer 3's concerns about study "feasibility" and ability "to identify an impact" were based on confusion about the study's primary outcome and the idea that it is rare. Having any fall is, unfortunately, a common experience in State Veterans Homes.

   This study has adequate power to detect a difference in any fall. We powered the study to have 90% power using an alpha of 0.01 to detect an improvement from 50% to 40% (F.4.d.), a smaller improvement than in other fall prevention studies.

   Concerns about underreporting of falls and "potential bias towards the null" (Reviewer 2) are also reduced since we now clearly indicate that our primary outcome was always the broad category of any fall. Any fall is less sensitive to underreporting, because it is not affected by the absolute number of falls and reduces selection bias. To check for underreporting, we will, as Reviewer 2 suggests, look at trends among all reported outcomes to see if there are increases in other outcomes over the study period (F.3.a.).

   "Concern about...duration of post-implementation [period]" (Summary point 4; Reviewers 2 & 3).

> We carefully analyzed our overall study timeline and are now able to perform 12-month sustainment evaluations for both Waves 1 and 2 with the same number of sites as in the original submission (n = 8) by shortening the adaptation period. The intervention period consequently now ends one quarter later than in the original submission. Nevertheless, the limited data collection from each site during the final 6 months gives us sufficient time to analyze the bulk of the qualitative data. This longer follow-up period strengthens the study's assessment of sustainability and, consequently, the study impact. To accommodate these changes and others made in response to reviewer suggestions, we increased year 4's budget...

How do you like these two response documents? Differing page limits influenced the amount of detail. Did the brief version still convince? Did the longer version maintain interest? How would you respond in similar circumstances?

References

Elliot, A. J. (2006). The Hierarchical Model of Approach-Avoidance Motivation. *Motiv Emot, 30*, 111–116. https://doi.org/10.1007/s11031-006-9028-7

Heath, C., & Heath, D. (2010). *Switch: How to Change When Change is Hard*. Random House.

Chapter 14
Cutting and Editing

Cutting text is difficult. Tight deadlines make it stressful. I have experience with that. All my colleagues know about the time I misremembered a proposal's page limit, leading to panicked edits hours before submission.

The root of my mistake lay in the funding organization's reduction of the maximum page count. Between my first submission and resubmission, the total count decreased from 25 pages (a one-page overview plus 24 pages of narrative text) to 15 pages (the overview plus 14 pages of narrative). For my reapplication, I struggled with the new constraints. Draft after draft, the page count dropped, but only incrementally. I found cutting hard partly because the old 25-page limit floated in my head like the ghost of a beautiful idea.

So I began chanting one number, 15, to drive the phantom from my mind. Unfortunately, at some point, I started attributing 15 pages to the narrative section alone, meaning I thought I had one more page than I did.

Hours before the deadline, my proposal had a one-page overview and 15—instead of 14—narrative pages. I did not notice the mistake. I was proud of having successfully crafted a concise application so much shorter than the original. Then, in my final check, I realized my error.

Being one page over the limit for the narrative section meant the grant would be automatically rejected once received. I had to eliminate a full page. But that seemed impossible. How could I delete so much from a proposal already pared down to its essential elements?

Fear motivated me. With a ticking clock and a pounding heart, I cut, radically applying a scalpel to every paragraph. I wiped out words, phrases, and sentences.

At the end of two hours, I had a new version, one page shorter. And to my surprise, it was not demonstrably worse. It made the same points. My arguments were still clear. And the proposal was subsequently funded.

Through that experience, I learned a valuable lesson. No matter how compressed a text is, cutting is *always* possible.

C. W. Hartmann, *Grant Writing Fundamentals Made Easy*,
https://doi.org/10.1007/978-3-032-35723-6_14

14.1 Principles for Cutting Text

Many techniques for editing concentrate on minutiae. When a text is far over a limit, this may feel counterintuitive. Why fixate on trivial things when you have big issues? But there is a saying in the ultralight hiking world, "Pay attention to the ounces, and the pounds will take care of themselves." Think of your manuscript as a backpack. Your job is to throw out even the tiniest nonessential items. This will eventually reduce the overall weight.

Cutting text-based ounces may require grammatical editing. If you struggle with grammar or need a refresher, I recommend searching online for Purdue University's On-campus Writing Lab (Purdue Owl, 2026). They have posts on verbs, adjectives, participles, clauses... you name it. Their site covers the writing process, punctuation, editing, and more. If you want to dig deeper into editing your own work, pick up Roy Peter Clark's *Writing Tools: 50 Essential Strategies for Every Writer* (2008). If you feel boxed in by grammatical rules, check out Verlyn Klinkenborg's *Several Short Sentences about Writing* (2012). If you write from an underrepresented perspective, you might enjoy Deepa Anappara and Taymour Soomro's *Letters to a Writer of Color* (2023) or Felicia Rose Chavez's *The Anti-Racist Writing Workshop: How to Decolonize the Creative Classroom* (2021) for support in developing your own writing style.

Several principles guide effective cutting. When employing these, keep in mind the funding organization's character, word, or page limits. Most organizations have mechanisms for weeding out applications that do not comply with requirements. Ignoring their policies is often automatic grounds for rejection. So even if you find a sneaky way to circumvent a rule, keep its spirit in mind and err on the side of caution.

Editing should be the first recourse. Yes, you may be able to "gain" a few lines by choosing to artificially hyphenate words. Sometimes, you can manipulate formatting and still remain within guidelines. But these techniques target the wrong bullseye. They presuppose that all existing words are so important that you cannot delete any of them. As my story above shows, that is not true. Every proposal contains superfluous or redundant parts and often benefits from cutting to home in on the most important points.

Reviewers' needs drive edits. In everything you do to decrease the length of an application, also remember the reviewer. Many non-editing-based techniques *reduce* the quality of a reviewer's reading experience. Do not squeeze paragraphs together without space between them. Reading dense text creates cognitive strain. For the same reason, avoid shrinking the text in graphics beyond the suggested limit (usually, no smaller than the equivalent of nine-point font). Think before deleting graphics entirely, particularly if they succinctly explain critical information and help to create visual pauses. (See Chap. 11, Sect. 11.7 for more about graphics.) Resist the temptation to develop new abbreviations. These are typically easy for only one person: you (see Chap. 7, Sect. 7.6).

No grant is so perfect that it cannot be shortened through careful editing.

14.2 Read Aloud

One of the best ways to edit is to read aloud. If you have not tried it, you might not believe how well it works. The next time you write a formal document, find a private space and speak the document to an invisible audience or have a software program or app read it to you. Mark every phrase you stumble over, paragraphs you have to read or listen to twice, typos an autocorrect program did not pick up. Note where points repeat or sentences are so long you must catch your breath in the middle. Admit that some passages bore you.

The brain hears spoken words differently than those it reads silently. When you hear a proposal through your ears, it is as though you encounter it for the first time. You have greater difficulty glossing over mistakes, awkward wording or construction, and logic problems. If you use software to listen to what you wrote, change the voice or the reading speed to prevent your brain from slumping into low gear. You will be surprised by what you catch.

14.3 Construct Simple Sentences

The last time most of us took a class that emphasized English writing was in high school. The teachers taught us to vary sentence structure, use long introductory clauses, and to never split an infinitive (like I did here). We learned how to use words such as "however," "therefore," and "regardless." And teachers advised us never to begin a sentence with a conjunction (and, but, or, yet, etc.). We impressed these instructors by following those directions. After all, simple sentences were what we wrote in elementary school.

You may think, "I've gotten this far with my writing the way it is. Why change now?" But when you write a grant, you sell your ideas for money. The people standing between you and that money are the reviewers. Often, making the reviewer's job as simple and painless as possible means putting aside what you learned in high school. The first hurdle is sentence structure. Simple *is* better.

I have written many proposals in which every sentence follows a subject–verb–object structure. These simply constructed sentences do not have to be short. And they do not have to be similar sounding. The initial two paragraphs of Chap. 1 contain sentences of varying lengths, some short, others not, each sounding different. Repetition and similarity lead to boredom. *Simplicity*, in its infinite variations, engages a reader while making the task of reading effortless.

Exercise: Simple Sentences

For each of the following A-B pairs, jot down or say aloud which you find easier to read, A or B.

Pair One

A. Because the literature on high-reliability organizations emphasizes the necessity of a "preoccupation with failure" and the importance of a highly uniform safety climate, [our survey] instrument is scored to reflect the percentage of "problematic responses"—answers that suggest an absence of safety climate. (Hartmann et al., 2008)

B. The literature on high reliability organizations emphasizes the necessity of a "preoccupation with failure" and the importance of a highly uniform safety climate. We therefore scored our survey instrument to reflect the percentage of "problematic responses"—answers that suggest an *absence* of safety climate.

Pair Two

A. Although previous studies have shown that the intervention did cause users to believe they received worse care, by pointing out deficiencies in the quality of their care, data are needed to more fully understand the potential effects of such an intervention, in particular, how the intervention can impact doctor–patient communication. (Hartmann et al., 2007)

B. Previous studies showed that users believed they received worse care when an intervention pointed out deficiencies in the quality of their care. We therefore need more data to understand the potential effects of interventions such as this one. Specifically, our understanding would benefit from knowing how this type of intervention can affect doctor–patient communication.

The A examples are from my early published work (mea culpa!). Likely, you found the B examples easier to read, regardless of the content. In the B examples, each sentence is structured as subject–verb–object.

Review a recent piece of your own writing. Search for sentences that do not have the subject and verb at the beginning. Can you rework them? If you want help, use one of numerous apps focused on identifying needlessly complex writing. If you do not have examples from your own work, choose literature in your field or from your organization. Dissect the sentences. What would you improve?

14.4 Edit for Easier Reading

Proposal writers need not be editing experts. But, as William Zinsser says in the Introduction to his book *On Writing Well* (2006, p. xii), "[T]he essence of writing is rewriting. Just because [you]'re writing fluently doesn't mean [you]'re writing well." Below are four editing tips that not only improve writing style but also help cut space.

Take out words you added for emphasis. Remove words and phrases such as "importantly," "surprisingly," "notably," "of primary importance," "of note," etc. You probably inserted these to help the reviewer see what is important, surprising, notable... But this does not work. Instead, accomplish that goal through clear organization with the 1-3-2 principle. (See Chap. 7, Sect. 7.1) Using these words and phrases also lulls you into feeling you do not need to present points in the most compelling language possible, which is incorrect. Additionally, in the worst case, emphatic wording annoys a reviewer because it implies they cannot decide on an opinion themselves. Instead, let a reviewer draw their own conclusions from facts and your spin (see Chap. 11, Sect. 11.1 for more on the importance of spin).

Remove unnecessary introductions. A grant writer has a goal for each section and paragraph. A desire to state this goal directly leads to sentences such as, "The next section will describe our prior work" or "This paragraph will discuss some of the known conflicts in the field and how we address them." To save space, cut this type of superfluous text and, instead, orient the reviewer using first sentences and headings that focus on main messages. Here are example improvements to the above introductory phrases: "Prior work underscores our mastery of essential methods" or "The research design addresses known conflicts in the field by incorporating [list specifics here]."

Tone down big words. In the spirit of simplicity, avoid using big words or longer phrases when simple, short alternatives exist. "Utilize" becomes "use." "Endeavor" becomes "try." "Proficiency" becomes "skill." Enlist AI to analyze your text and find alternatives. Big words do not make you sound smart. They make reading more difficult.

Eliminate "that." Sometimes, do you not need the word "that" in a sentence. How do you tell? Read the sentence aloud *without* the "that." If it still makes sense, take it out. You will find [that] sentences flow more smoothly.

14.5 Ten Tips for Cutting

Here is a procedure that incorporates ten successful methods for reducing the length of a proposal, assuming you have already cut what you can and used the techniques above. I call this procedure scalpel editing. It might be painful. But it is effective. You can employ these at any point in the writing process. I present them in rough order of priority, beginning with what is easiest and assists most. I suggest moving through them successively, only employing the later tips when you run out of other options.

14.5.1 Read for Logic

Begin by scanning your headings and subheadings, particularly in the background-providing section. Do they tell the full story of your application? Do they make logical sense in the order they are written? This critical assessment provides an opportunity to evaluate whether you have too much or not enough of what you need. You might initially add more text when you do this, if you find something is missing. But as you evaluate for logic, simultaneously evaluate whether you require everything you wrote. Does every sentence and paragraph add something new? Do you exceed the amount of detail required for a reviewer to grasp your point? Does the submission needlessly flaunt what you know or, instead, efficiently convince and move on? Are your arguments pertinent to reviewer and funding organization priorities or do they digress? Anything that does not bolster the application's foundational arguments wastes space.

14.5.2 Read for Redundancy

We often write proposal sections at various times. Sometimes sections are written by different people. These things can lead to redundancy. A simple and relatively painless way to identify this involves putting your application aside for as long as possible (at least a day is helpful, but do what works for your timeline). Then, scrutinize it with an eye for where you say the same thing twice. Can you refer a reader to a prior section where you already made the point, paraphrase the message, or cut?

In rare instances, repetition may be necessary. But think about where you place the information. Follow the 1-3-2 principle (see Chap. 7, Sect. 7.1). Move it to where it has the greatest effect.

14.5.3 Focus on Sections That Are Disproportionately Long

After employing the techniques above, if your text is still too long, you need to dig into editing. Begin where it is both necessary and easiest. Choose sections that stand out for being longer than others. If your project has three aims, for example, and (without a justifiable reason) the methods for Aim 1 are a page longer than the methods for Aims 2 and 3, begin with the Aim 1 methods section. An application that lacks reasonable balance implies the author knows less about some things than others. Reviewers may perceive you as an expert on Aim 1 methods but think you have a weaker understanding of what you propose for Aims 2 and 3. Cut to achieve logical consistency in length.

14.5.4 Watch for Blank Lines

If you find empty space at the bottom of a page or elsewhere, manipulate the text to eliminate it. These gaps might be the result of ill-placed graphics. Electronic documents also like to keep paragraphs together with a default function called "window/orphan control." Try turning off this setting for the entire document. If your technological needs exceed your abilities, search online for information about your issue or ask AI.

14.5.5 Wrap Text Around Graphics

Instead of having blank space next to a graphic, wrap text around one side. But it sometimes makes more sense to prioritize cognitive ease. If wrapping creates a narrow column

> where you
> read only
> a few
> words at
> a time,

cognitive strain results. Avoid this and *enlarge* the graphic so it spans an entire page, knowing you will save room with other techniques.

14.5.6 Look for Paragraphs Where Several Words Wrap Down Onto the Next Line

I call this the "paragraph bump method." It involves relatively little editing. Go through the offending paragraph and tighten your language until the final words move up to the previous line. This gives you one extra line on the page. Find all the paragraphs in your document where this is the case. The more desperate you are, the more bloodthirsty you need to be about implementing this technique. AI can help with this. I first target paragraphs with only a few words on the subsequent line. If that does not give me the space I require, I address those that have half a line of dangling words.

14.5.7 Reduce Spacing Between Paragraphs

Having white space in a proposal makes reading easier. But white space takes up room. Adjust spacing and paragraph formatting to reduce (not eliminate) white space. Preserve the visual effect. A tiny white area is better than none.

14.5.8 Reorganize Prepositional Phrases, Particularly Those That Repeat

We often use prepositional phrases without awareness, especially those related to our work. I conduct my research in nursing homes, so I write about "staff in nursing homes" or "research in nursing homes." But both these phrases can be shortened:

"nursing home staff" and "nursing home research." A surprising number of prepositional phrases can be changed. Be vigilant as you write or edit. Use an automatic search and replace function or enlist AI's help. You save an "ounce" every time you do this; within a longer proposal, these ounces add up.

14.5.9 Make Each Paragraph Bump Up One Line

This version of the paragraph bump method builds on the technique in Sect. 14.5.6 and requires courage and commitment. Begin at the top of the application. Shorten the word count of *every* paragraph until it is at least one entire line shorter. (For example, count how many lines this paragraph occupies and imagine cutting until it has one fewer.)

Treat all paragraphs equally. That may be difficult, especially since you have already used this technique before. But stick to it. Avoid allowing any paragraph a pass. Take consolation from the fact that all writing benefits from rigorous editing. What is left behind will be clearer for having less unnecessary information. If worry about "losing" your words forever prevents you from implementing this step, create a separate document to store what you remove. Then, attack every paragraph.

14.5.10 Use Technique #9 Again

As painful as it sounds, if your application is still too long, you must repeat the technique in Sect. 14.5.9. Impossible, you say? Possible, I reply. The intention to discover new places to squeeze is driven by desperation and determination. Whenever I think my text is as tight as it can be, that each word is necessary, I always find something to change. I start again from the beginning and implement my editing skills ruthlessly. This is why I call it scalpel editing. Instead of feeling sorry for this section or that one, I develop an egalitarian remorselessness.

14.6 Practice Editing Every Day

Marketing professionals spend their careers studying how to craft compelling emails because they want to sell something to someone who is not necessarily interested. Proposals can feel that way too—they pitch your project to a tired but well-meaning reviewer. Daily email offers an opportunity to practice editing and improve your ability to pitch your ideas. Like proposal text, most email text (even that generated by AI) can improve. Here are email editing techniques that will help with proposal writing. These techniques relate to what Chap. 7 describes for promoting a reader's cognitive ease.

With AI helping draft emails at an increasing frequency, you may be tempted to skip this information. You might not write many emails yourself, accepting instead the suggestions AI populates. But even the text generated by AI can get better (see Chap. 14, Sect. 14.7). I encourage you to read on, because the less you participate in editing, the more difficult writing a grant is.

Exercise: Find Buried Messages
Read the email below. Find the main points from the perspective of the recipient. Highlight these or say them aloud.

> We are adding users to our IncrediApp and your name is on our list. IncrediApp provides deidentified information about our company's community to assist with management decisions. Although we expect most people will want to take advantage of this great opportunity, if you would not like to be added to the IncrediApp application, please respond to this email with a request to be taken off the list. We would like to have all responses by the end of business on June 24. We are communicating this to everyone, because anyone with access to the IncrediApp application will eventually need approval, which will involve some easy interface with us, the roll-out team, through a few emails that you will see. We don't want there to be any confusion when emails are sent to users, so please let us know your preference.

Following the 1-3-2 principle (see Chap. 7, Sect.7.1), what would be a better first sentence for the email? Write it down or say it aloud. How would you present the remaining information? Would you use text, bullets, or a table? What do you think will engage readers and achieve you the response you desire?

I imagine the author of the above email wrote the sentences as they thought of them. But ideas as they occur to us are often jumbled. We do not think in 1-3-2. The difference between an okay email and an excellent one is often whether the author has taken time to edit. Below is an example revision.

Please reply to this email by June 24 if you would like to be removed from the roll-out list for IncrediApp. You are currently on our list.

- *IncrediApp assists with management decisions by providing deidentified information about our company's community.*
- *Anyone with access to IncrediApp will eventually need approval through easy interface with the roll-out team via email.*
- *To limit the roll-out to only interested participants, please* ***respond by June 24 if you are not interested and want to be removed from the roll-out list****.*

14.6.1 Remove Redundancy

Email is a great place to notice how often we repeat ourselves. Below is an email example. Where is it repetitive?

We are cancelling all co-investigator calls for the summer (June, July, and August) and will start our co-investigator calls again in September. I sent meeting cancellations. There is not much happening with the study in the summer, and we do not want to take up your valuable time.

Although I sent out meeting cancellations for each of these meetings, I also wanted to send out this informational email to let everyone know what was going on and when we would have our next meeting.

To the author, the second paragraph probably seemed helpful when they wrote it. As a reader, do you think it adds much to the first? When you got to the bottom and figured out you read a second paragraph that told you nothing new, were you confused or annoyed? How would you eliminate the repetition? Here is one revision.

You received meeting cancellation notices for the next three co-investigator calls (June, July, and August) because there is not much happening with the study in these months. Enjoy the summer and see you on the September call.

Catching your own repetition in a proposal is difficult without practice. Email represents fertile ground to hone that skill.

14.6.2 Be Brief

One of email's core qualities is the reader's expectation of brevity. To adhere to this expectation, condense phrasing, eliminate unnecessary words, and sharpen points. To practice further, limit yourself to one main message per email. Lead with that and only add text if it contains new information. If you have a lot of news to report, decide whether to employ bullets or even break the email apart, sending multiple messages instead. Test important emails on people who represent your potential audience. Then, apply these stronger editing skills to your next grant.

14.6.3 Eliminate Unknown Words

Chapter 7, Section 7.6 explains why abbreviations frustrate reviewers. Here is a real-life example of an email subject line.

"Subject: PMDB changes r/t WBRA"

When I received this, the only word I understood was "changes."* You might think a recipient appreciates abbreviations because they help keep content brief. But beware. Just like in proposal writing, include only those you are *sure* the recipient will understand without a moment of hesitation. Anything else can backfire. Becoming comfortable with catching and eliminating abbreviations in email will help you feel the same way when you write a proposal.

*Here are what those acronyms meant: PMDB = prevention and management of disruptive behavior class, r/t = related to, and WBRA = workplace behavior risk assessment.

14.6.4 Remember Your Audience

The more your audience is on your mind as you write your daily emails, the more your reviewers will be on your mind as you prepare an application. Your choice of language and tone is linked to your readers. Is the audience for an email a boss? A friend? Five thousand people you never met? What do you know about them? How much do they know about your subject? Anticipate their needs. Use language they understand. And, recipient or reviewer, respect their time.

14.7 Example of Human Versus AI for Editing and Cutting

As noted in Chap. 1, Section 1.3, at the suggestion of the publisher, I used AI copyediting software to edit this book before publication. Of course, after using it, I did everything I suggest you do. I checked its work and accepted only what I thought improved the text. In general, it was a straightforward process.

Copyediting by a dedicated copyediting AI software program is different from content generation. It is also different from asking a general AI software program to edit. In addition, in proposal writing, text AI generates or changes may be different from material that convinces reviewers. If you use AI at all, regularly review funding organization restrictions on its use (for more on this, see Chap. 1, Sect. 1.3).

To investigate a general AI software's editing capabilities at the time of writing this book, I asked AI (ChatGPT 5.1) to edit a paragraph from an early draft of one of my funded scientific proposals (with only the citations eliminated). The paragraph describes the conceptual framework we used for the study. The intervention we used is called the "LOCK program," so you will see that referenced in the paragraphs below. The LOCK program is a nursing home clinical care intervention that uses brief, stand-up meetings of frontline staff to improve quality of care. The grant was submitted to and funded by the US National Institute on Aging.

14.7.1 Initial Early Draft Version

> The adoption of evidence-based interventions into practice suffers from a significant, documented time lag. This is of potentially even greater concern in nursing homes, where adoption requires surmounting additional hurdles. Analyzing and overcoming barriers to more rapid adoption, as well as identifying facilitators, thus represents an important mechanism for promoting improvements in care. Relational coordination is an evidence-based framework for studying and implementing high performance. In our study, it undergirds the primary intervention, the LOCK program. Relational coordination emphasizes that staff across all job types must be connected by high-quality interactions to create an environment in which teams achieve top outcomes. Healthcare organizations with high relational coordination have been shown to achieve higher quality of care, lower postoperative pain, higher quality of postoperative functioning, shorter length of stay, and higher patient satisfaction and quality

of life. And despite the documented importance of undisrupted sleep, no study we know of addresses sleep improvement for nursing home residents using an intervention to improve staff members' relational coordination.

The following is AI's edited version, followed by the text from the submitted grant (written by humans). I asked AI to include its reasoning for any edits. So I also went back after the fact and wrote in my thoughts about the reasoning behind the changes for the final, submitted version. See what you think.

14.7.2 *AI Edits to the Initial Draft Version, with Reasons*

This is the prompt I used when I asked AI to edit. "Edit the paragraph below about a pragmatic clinical trial's conceptual framework. The paragraph is part of a grant application to the US National Institute on Aging. The LOCK program mentioned is an intervention that uses brief, stand-up meetings of nursing home frontline staff. Do not add any new facts. Focus on editing. Tighten/rewrite/reorder the text, improve the logic, and make the content and structure maximally persuasive for US National Institutes of Health grant reviewers. Provide the reasoning for any changes you make."

This is what AI produced, in approximately one second.

> The adoption of evidence-based interventions into routine practice is notoriously slow, and this lag is especially pronounced in nursing homes, where implementation must overcome additional operational and organizational barriers. Understanding and addressing these barriers—as well as the factors that facilitate uptake—is therefore essential to accelerating improvements in care. Relational coordination, an evidence-based framework for achieving high performance, provides the conceptual foundation for our primary intervention, the LOCK program, which uses brief, stand-up frontline staff meetings to strengthen team functioning. Relational coordination posits that high-quality communication and relationships among staff across all roles are critical for achieving optimal outcomes. Organizations with stronger relational coordination consistently demonstrate higher quality of care, lower postoperative pain, better postoperative functioning, shorter lengths of stay, and greater patient satisfaction and quality of life. Yet despite the well-established importance of uninterrupted sleep in nursing home residents, no prior study to our knowledge has attempted to improve resident sleep by enhancing staff relational coordination—highlighting both the novelty and potential impact of the proposed work (OpenAI, 2025).

These are the AI-generated reasons for its edits.

1. Strengthened logical flow
   - Original text jumped from the adoption gap → nursing homes → barriers → relational coordination with only loose transitions.
   - Revised version creates a clear, persuasive progression:
     1. The problem: slow adoption.
     2. Why it matters more in nursing homes.
     3. The need to understand barriers/facilitators.

    4. Introduction of relational coordination as the solution framework.
    5. Its evidence base.
    6. The gap this study fills (sleep).

2. Improved clarity and concision

    - Removed redundancies (e.g., "represents an important mechanism for facilitating improvements in care").
    - Combined related concepts to avoid fragmentation and repetitive sentence structure.

3. Stronger positioning of relational coordination

    - Moved relational coordination earlier and integrated it more directly with the intervention (LOCK).
    - Tightened its definition for reviewers who may not be experts but want clarity fast.

4. Enhanced persuasiveness

    - Framed relational coordination findings as "consistent" rather than listing outcomes abruptly.
    - Highlighted the *novelty* of integrating relational coordination to improve sleep—critical for significance sections.

5. Addressed reviewer expectations

    - Explicitly tied conceptual framework → intervention → expected mechanism → innovation.
    - Ensured each sentence advances significance or rationale rather than describing background passively (OpenAI, 2025).

14.7.3 Final, Submitted Paragraph, with Reasons

This is the paragraph from the funded grant.

> The adoption of evidence-based interventions into practice suffers from a significant, documented time lag. This is of potentially even greater concern in nursing homes, where adoption requires surmounting nursing home staffing issues, resource concerns, and traditional top-down approaches to quality improvement. Relational coordination is an evidence-based framework emphasizing that staff across all job types must be connected by high-quality interactions and supportive relationships to create an environment in which teams achieve improved outcomes. Healthcare organizations—including nursing homes—with high relational coordination achieve higher quality of care, lower postoperative pain, higher quality of postoperative functioning, shorter length of stay, and higher patient satisfaction and quality of life. In our study, relational coordination undergirds the primary intervention: the LOCK program applied to sleep.

Here are my post hoc reasons for the edits that resulted in this final version. I wrote these before looking at the AI output.

1. *Implement the 1-3-2 principle* (Chap. 7, Sect. 7.1). The edited version keeps the initial (the "1" position) sentence because it expresses an idea common across all research about furthering change within a system. Many reviewers should resonate with this fact. The final (the "2" position) sentence in the early draft focused on explicating a knowledge gap. Instead, as editing progressed, our team decided it was more important to end with the fact that relational coordination grounds the proposed work, particularly because the phrase relational coordination otherwise only appears in the middle of the paragraph (the "3" position).
2. *Emphasize showing, not telling* (Chap. 7, Sect. 7.5). The early draft includes numerous sentences that state information without providing facts to back them up. The final version addresses this by consolidating main points, emphasizing examples that support the claims.
3. *Condense for brevity and clarity*. We shortened the text significantly to save space and tighten language. We also eliminated redundancy with the rest of the application: removed information about proposal methods (identifying barriers and facilitators) and the importance of uninterrupted sleep. The final version highlights the key points that describe the framework and how it was used by other organizations to improve outcomes.

14.7.4 Thoughts on AI and Human Versions

As you know, no piece of writing is perfect. When I looked back after a few years at the final, submitted paragraph, I found things I would change. I still think the first sentence packs punch and is potentially engaging for reviewers from various disciplines. But a different sentence that immediately introduces the concept of relational coordination might be better. I like AI's sentence about the outcomes other healthcare organizations experienced using relational coordination. If there were enough space, that might be a better first sentence than the equivalent one from the final version. And yet…

AI's narrative has significant flaws. First, it violates the principle of writing without extraneous phrasing. This does not surprise me. AI creates its own understanding of how to write a grant based on what it can access. The examples it collects may not represent the strongest writing. As documented extensively in this book, reviewers benefit from clarity and an approach to cognitive ease (see Chap. 1, Sect. 1.1) that supports rapid assimilation of information. Long sentence structure does not do that. I therefore disagree with AI's choice to combine "related concepts to avoid fragmentation." AI does not get tired when reading. Reviewers do.

Second, AI needlessly adds pretentious words: "posit" instead of "is," "optimal" instead of "top" or "improved." It also included the superfluous phrase, "highlighting both the novelty and potential impact of the proposed work," which tells the reviewer what to think. A better strategy involves letting the reviewer determine novelty and impact based on what they read. A well-organized proposal never needs to insert such words, instead enabling a reviewer to draw these conclusions on their own.

Finally, the AI version contains dangerous inaccuracies. It changed, "This [lag] is of potentially even greater concern in nursing homes" to "this lag is especially pronounced in nursing homes." The difference is subtle but important. The former statement does not need a citation—it is conjecture based on presented facts and can stand alone as such. The AI version states a fact, "more pronounced," that needs a citation. But that citation does not exist because the fact is fabricated and untrue.

In addition, it changed "an important mechanism for facilitating improvements" to "therefore essential to accelerating improvements." Again, this represents not only a change in meaning but also a dangerous change in veracity. And AI praises itself for the addition of the word "consistently" in the sentence about organizations with higher relational coordination demonstrating higher quality of care. But it added the word without knowing whether that statement is supported in the literature.

In other words, in many places within this short paragraph, AI chose to invent facts despite a direct prompt to avoid this ("do not add any new facts").

When I ran this experiment, I did not know how it would turn out. The results gave me pause. I had a good experience using AI when copyediting this book. But that was with a copyediting-specific software program, not a general large-language-model like ChatGPT. If I were actually using AI to edit a paragraph to include in a grant, I would go back-and-forth with it about its product. I might give it some example text from the current proposal or from previous ones so that it has a better idea of my style. I would be more specific in my prompts. I would certainly scrutinize the results for errors and ask AI to learn from its mistakes.

I believe that if a person has a longer conversation with AI, the quality of the final product will improve. AI is fast, up at any hour, and willing to revise ad nauseam. But I also know it is imperfect, as are we. Ultimately, I believe humans must lean into our own capabilities for critical thinking, writing, and editing to craft—alone or with AI—the best proposal possible.

References

Anappara, D., & Soomro, T. (Eds.). (2023). *Letters to a Writer of Color*. Random House.

Chavez, F. R. (2021). *The Anti-Racist Writing Workshop: How to Decolonize the Creative Classroom*. Haymarket Books.

Clark, R. P. (2008). *Writing Tools: 50 Essential Strategies for Every Writer*. Little, Brown and Company.

Hartmann, C. W., Rosen, A. K., Meterko, M., Shokeen, P., Zhao, S., Singer, S., Falwell, A., & Gaba, D. M. (2008). An overview of patient safety climate in the VA. *Health Services Research, 43*(4), 1263–1284. https://doi.org/10.1111/j.1475-6773.2008.00839.x

Hartmann C. W., Sciamanna C. N., Blanch D. C., Mui S., Lawless H., Manocchia M., Rosen R. K., Pietropaoli A. (2007). A website to improve asthma care by suggesting patient questions for physicians: qualitative analysis of user experiences. *Journal of Medical Internet Research, 9*(1):e3. https://doi.org/10.2196/jmir.9.1.e3

Klinkenborg, V. (2012). *Several Short Sentences About Writing*. Knopf.
OpenAI. (2025). ChatGPT (5.1 version) [Large language model]. https://chat.openai.com/chat
Purdue Owl–Purdue University. (2026). https://owl.purdue.edu/
Zinsser, W. (2006). *On Writing Well*. Harper Collins.

Chapter 15
What to Do After a Grant Is Funded

15.1 Keeping Good Records of Grant Applications

Your participation in a grant submission, whether as the principal investigator or in another role, is part of your career history. Because of that, someone will eventually want to know details. If you have a lengthy career, you will have a long list of grants in which you participate. Avoid thinking that you will remember everything, that others will help you remember, or that an electronic file system will enable you to unearth information about each submission quickly.

Instead, create a grant tracking mechanism. Include all submitted grants, funded or not, regardless of your role. Aside from my curriculum vitae, this is the document I access and update the most.

The following bulleted list is what I have learned to record. I suggest you use Excel or a similar spreadsheet program to make a table that contains this information, although Word or something like it will do in a pinch. The list may seem too long. But at some point, I have been asked for or wanted every piece of information here. Below, I also suggest items for which you can keep a running total (another reason why Excel is better). Create a row for each submission (not just the funded projects). The items below are column headers.

- Submission date
- Grant type
- Funding organization
- Your role on the grant
- Name of principal investigator (if not you)
- Submission number (first submission, first resubmission, etc.)
- Name or number of study section or review panel to which grant was assigned
- Score
- Result (funded or not)
- Project acronym (if applicable)
- Title submitted with grant application

C. W. Hartmann, *Grant Writing Fundamentals Made Easy*,
https://doi.org/10.1007/978-3-032-35723-6_15

- Award number (formal number assigned to grant by funding organization)
- Institutional project number (if applicable)
- Amount of full budget
- Amount of each budget year
- Your percent effort on the grant (by year if the percent varies)
- Official start and end dates of the grant (if the grant is funded)
- Institutional Review Board title (if applicable and different from grant title)

I bold the rows for grants that are funded, making them easier to recognize. At some point, you are likely to want cumulative data. I suggest you create formulas to total the following at the bottom of your spreadsheet

- Number of grants funded with you as principal investigator (including mentored career development or other career awards for yourself).
- Funding amount you receive as principal investigator (use the full budget amount to calculate total).
- Number of grants funded with you as co-investigator.
- Funding amount for grants with you as co-investigator (also use the full budget amount—give yourself credit for being on the team that got the full amount).

Making such a spreadsheet is easy. Update it whenever you or someone else submits a proposal and when you receive notification about the outcome. If you already have several funded grants, it might be time consuming to populate initially. But you will pat yourself on the back when someone asks you for this information later or you must sing your own praises in a performance appraisal. If grants are part of your world, you need this database. Think of it as a necessary counterpart to your curriculum vitae.

15.2 Unexpected Changes Post Award

There are often many months between a submission and the notice that a grant was awarded. In those months, life moves ahead. Plans for project management evolve. People named in your application may no longer be able to participate in the work. The budget might need adjustment due to increases in prices, unanticipated raises, or movement of personnel. Individuals switch departments or institutions. The list for what can change is long. Rest assured that those in charge of managing grants, both at your institution and at the funding organization, are familiar with the processes necessary to help you respond appropriately.

Many funding institutions allow grant award recipients some leeway in how they run a project and allocate funds. Circumstances requiring prior approval are usually clearly indicated. For most funding organizations, significant post-application/pre-award changes require formal authorization through a project modification process. This ensures regulatory compliance and that the modifications align with the approved proposal.

If you are unsure, contact a grants administrator at your home institution. This person, or someone they put you in contact with, will help you assess the extent of a change and what to do. They may be willing to look at drafts of the documents you need to submit. They will also likely recommend that you contact the individual in charge of your grant at the funding organization. That person will know the regulations and how to access required forms.

Never delay contacting someone because you are afraid of the unknown. The earlier you engage with individuals who know answers, the more time you will have to prepare your documentation and arguments. After working hard on your proposal, tackling yet another administrative hurdle may feel daunting. But these hurdles are put in place to keep everyone aware and informed. In the end, you benefit from clarifying your plans with the funding organization because it enables them to trust and support you as your project progresses.

15.3 Guidelines for Manuscript Authorship and Project Data Use

One of my teams' most frequently requested templates is our publication and data use guidelines for grants. This is because discussions about publication authorship and use of data can be challenging to have with colleagues. Academia has a "publish or perish" reputation, where not every authorship position is viewed equally. And people can feel proprietary about data. This may generate strong emotions and jockeying for coveted spots or access. Early career faculty and researchers may have difficulty navigating these discussions or pushing forward their own needs. A document generated by the entire team at the start of a project can help.

The document presents a structure. But equally important is the *process* by which a team generates the final version. That process usually involves anyone on the project who has a possibility of authorship. This includes principal investigators, co-investigators, fellows, trainees, and staff. Only you and your team will know the full list.

One suggested process for generating the final document is the following. Create an initial draft, preferably with consultation from the other principal investigators (if applicable), key co-investigators, or mentors. Send that document around via email or put it in a shared folder and invite people to comment. Revise it based on comments. Then develop a conversation guide (AI can help) to address issues about which individuals disagreed or topics that need further deliberation. (See Chap. 4, Sect. 4.5 for some ideas about how one can hold discussions.) Then, set up a meeting that is open to all affected team members and go through your guide.

If you know in advance that some subjects are likely to be thorny, state these during the meeting and have everyone *write down* their own answer first. This prevents individuals from dominating or swaying the conversation. Open the floor for comments and go around the room to hear from everyone, whether they speak up, put their comments in a chat, or send them to you privately. Reach consensus if possible. When people do not agree, state that the principal investigator(s) will communicate suggestions to the entire group.

In practice, these conversations are usually brief and easy to have. Because they happen at the beginning of a project, they also create a structure and process for future conversations. Since the final document is created with everyone's input, even early career principal investigators can then take a firm stand on subsequent issues if they arise.

The following box contains a draft template. It assumes two principal investigators and uses brackets for notes. It is only a guide. Modify it based on your own needs and circumstances. This should be a living document, so if people leave or join the team or there are other changes, revise it, have another discussion, and share the revision with the group.

Publication and Data Use Guidelines
[EXAMPLE project].

Publishing and other dissemination work for [EXAMPLE project] is critical. These publication and data use guidelines aim to maximize publications, fairness, generosity, and adherence to scientific authorship guidelines.

For purposes of this policy, [Drs. ABC and XYZ] are considered the principal investigators (PIs). [Drs. ABC and XYZ] have a long history of successful collaboration on studies. While it is ideal to involve both PIs in decisions pertaining to authorship, publication, and data use, sometimes only one of the PIs may be available. [Drs. ABC and XYZ] understand and agree that one of them can make decisions on behalf of both under such circumstances.

Affected Individuals

For purposes of this policy, the following individuals are considered co-investigators, collaborators, and other project team members (e.g., consultants, fellows, students, staff, etc.). [NOTE: You may want a different grouping or multiple groups. Include whomever you deem appropriate. It might be all people named in the grant or may only be those involved in a certain subpart of or supplement to the project. If you like, create different policies for various parts of the project. You can be explicit about how people make it onto this list, such as by attending meetings or filling key roles. You may want, here or below, to indicate how the project will manage team member transitions and papers coming from separate phases of the work. You might, for example, add a provision that if someone rotates off the project, they will still be considered a co-investigator, collaborator, or other project team member for a certain period for the purposes of publications and/or data use. You can also indicate what you will do if new individuals join the team.]

- [fill in with names and, if you like, roles].

Policies

1. All use of project-collected data must be approved by relevant Institutional Review Boards and by the project PIs.

2. Any individuals (co-investigators, collaborators, other project team members) interested in using project-collected data for publication or other use must inform the PIs via email and wait for PIs' approval before proceeding. [NOTE: You may wish to indicate PI(s) will also consult with or inform co-investigators before giving approval.]
3. Meetings with co-investigators, collaborators, and other project team members will be used as venues to gauge interest in publications and the use of data. Publication and data use discussions will occur at least quarterly in relevant meetings and more often when appropriate. [NOTE: You may wish to change how you have these discussions or get input, such as in shared documents.]
4. Co-investigators and collaborators will [always] be invited to participate in primary outcome papers of the project, if they meet authorship guidelines of the journal to which a manuscript is submitted. [NOTE: You might indicate that the PI(s) or a particular group will draft a list of papers that fulfill the study's objectives and identify people to lead these as well as the target journals.] The PIs, in conjunction with the first author of a relevant manuscript, will enable all co-investigators and collaborators opportunities to meet authorship criteria. (This is an opt-out type of policy for authorship.) [NOTE: You might indicate how you will "enable" this. Through email? Through announcements in meetings? In a shared document? You may also not want an "opt-out" policy but rather an "opt-in" policy, which would require different procedures.]
5. See #2 for the process for initiating other papers. Secondary papers authored by co-investigators or collaborators are encouraged (see #7 about first and last authorship). Such authorship will be discussed on regularly scheduled calls or, if moving quickly, by email or in a shared document. Interested participants should contact the PIs (see #1). [NOTE: You may want to add that these papers will be proposed by the PIs in a co-investigator-only forum first, so that open dialogue among co-investigators is possible before collaborators/other project team members are involved.]
6. Other project team members will be given opportunities to participate as authors of manuscripts as judged appropriate by the PI(s) and, if applicable, may become the first author of a specific manuscript. These other project team members must meet all criteria for authorship. Authorship for these other project team members will generally be by invitation only, but discussion of a paper may also be initiated by other project team members; see #2. (See #7 about first and last authorship.)
7. [Drs. ABC and XYZ] will be first and last authors on every project paper, unless they decline. [NOTE: You might wish to indicate a process by which you decide who is in what position, regardless of how many PIs are on the study.]
8. Authorship guidelines include involvement in the critical aspects of the project relevant to the paper, meaningful contribution to and review of drafts of the manuscript, review/approval of the final draft, and any other criteria set forth in journal guidelines.
9. The project team will maintain a list of planned/potential papers that includes the first and last authors, people interested in being co-authors in a tentative order, and the target journal(s). A tentative submission date will be established for each paper (the date to submit the manuscript for the first time to a specific journal).

10. The list of papers will be reviewed at least quarterly during regularly scheduled calls.
11. If the primary author of a manuscript does not/cannot move it toward submission in a timely fashion, the PIs have the right to reopen discussion of lead authorship and/or reschedule the timeline for submission.
12. Abstracts submitted to scientific meetings will follow the above guidelines, as applicable to the abstract format, including having the team develop a tentative list of abstracts as meeting submission deadlines approach.
13. All authors agree to use the "track changes" function [in a shared document] to edit a manuscript/abstract to facilitate transparency regarding the evolution of the manuscript/abstract and integration of comments.

15.4 Managing for Success

To get a driver's license, you must take a class and pass a test. Managing people is more complex than driving a car. Yet few graduate programs offer classes on how to manage others. Still, the success of your projects and career hinges partly on how well you do this.

15.4.1 Investigate What is Already Known

Do you have colleagues whom you admire for how they interact with others? Do they have low turnover among their staff? Do their staff seem happy, not just in their work life but in general? If you identify someone whose style you admire, set up a formal meeting to discuss their management philosophy.

Before you get together, do an online search or ask AI for help in finding reputable articles with advice for interviewing managers, characteristics of highly effective managers, and how to improve your management style. Develop your own set of questions, focusing on issues pertinent to you. Refine items after interviews as your needs shift and your experience increases.

As you investigate management best practices that fit with your requirements and style, always bear in mind your organization's human resources regulations. Know the lines that should not be crossed, stay within them, and ensure others do too. Being a good manager involves supporting success within your institution's parameters.

Free online courses in management are available. Also ask around your workplace. There might be seminars, workshops, or other opportunities, because organizations understand that better managers are more productive. And, of course, books on improving your management style abound. Choose those that fit your circumstances. When you search for books, look at lists developed by reputable sources. If you are a woman, note that many books on those lists are written by men, and probably *for* men, because while about half the US workforce is women, women are still mightily underrepresented in leadership positions. You might also search for books written by and for women leaders and managers. To obtain even more perspectives, search for lists and books written by and for other segments of the leadership and managerial workforce.

15.4.2 Consider an Evidence-Based Approach: Huddles

My team's management philosophy is grounded in the theory of relational coordination. As described by its inventor, Jody Hoffer Gittell in *High Performance Healthcare: Using the Power of Relationships to Achieve Quality, Efficiency and Resilience* (2009), this theory stresses the significance of communication and relationship building. At its core, it emphasizes the importance of frequent, timely, accurate, problem-solving (not blaming) communication that takes place in an atmosphere of shared goals, shared knowledge, and mutual respect.

You may wonder how a theory helps with the day-to-day operationalization of management practices. Yes, my teams and I set out to create the structures and processes that support core relational coordination principles. But how? One way is through huddling.

Huddles are brief, stand-up meetings focused on efficient information exchange. The term huddle is employed to distinguish these from longer meetings. There are many types of huddles. They are not a one-size-fits-all approach. You can find detailed information about huddles online. Ideal huddles share the characteristic that they create the *structure* to enable frequent, timely, and accurate communication.

Think about your work teams and times things did not go as planned or desired. Was having no regular way of communicating an underlying problem? Did information from various sectors come in too late to be useful? Was there a duplication of effort or a lack of awareness of what different people in the group were doing? Huddling can help with these issues.

Have a regular team huddle or institute this practice under times of stress. A huddle can be in person or virtual. It should start and stop on time. The facilitator should redirect distractions, acknowledge key information pieces, and develop group consensus around a clear action plan. A huddle should generally be 15 minutes at most. In that interval, the facilitator should check in with everyone present, asking them what they are working on and what they need help with. This energizes and coalesces a team and gives members knowledge to collaborate more effectively.

Huddles also benefit from the rigorous use of processes that support problem-solving communication focused on finding root causes for issues instead of blaming individuals. Processes include hearing from everyone using a "go around the room" technique, creating an action plan that is based on contributions of all people present, and ensuring that those most affected have the heaviest hand in defining and designing solutions. Do not expect perfection the first time or immediate buy-in from participants. Huddles might take a while to find their groove. Online searches and AI can identify ways to manage problems that arise and training on how to be a good huddle facilitator. Huddles provide both the structure for communication *and* the processes for sharing knowledge, developing shared goals, and growing mutual respect.

15.4.3 Avoid Negative Interactions

You spend many hours with your staff. Because you collaborate frequently, you may forget about the potentially lingering and detrimental effects of negative interactions, especially when you recognize a need for improvement. Under those circumstances, how you approach areas for potential growth may mark the difference between success and failure of a proposal submission or funded project.

With a good facilitator in place, huddles can provide a safe forum to address issues of concern because huddles focus on solving problems, not blaming people. Almost all problems have a systems-based component. This means that solutions might involve changing the systems within which people work. Huddles help avoid pointed discussions of individual failings and enable broader conversations about systems and mutual support. Huddles also actively and consistently focus on positive aspects of your team and its progress. Frequent huddles that everyone enjoys and benefits from foster an atmosphere of shared goals and mutual respect. When everyone feels part of a cohesive group, many subjects, even those potentially related to a specific individual, become easier to discuss as areas for *team* growth.

For concerns that require one-on-one conversations to guide someone toward a course correction or point out a mistake, sandwich that information between genuine, specific praise. Put praise first and last, making sure the positive feedback is honest and detailed. When I initially incorporated this technique, it felt counterintuitive. I thought problems should be addressed head-on, without preamble. Yes, they should be addressed. *And* you can *simultaneously* underscore where a person excels, how they are making progress, or the bigger picture in which the person is a key player. Very few people come to work intending to do a bad job. Recognize the larger context in which every individual operates and identify areas to support, particularly in the stressful context of preparing for a grant submission or executing a project.

15.4.4 Step Back from Anger

If you feel angry or otherwise negatively emotionally activated by an individual or situation, step back before acting. Draft what you want to say or write but avoid saying or sending it until you have calmed down and taken another look. Consider the potential effect of any negative things you contemplate doing. The person you are managing has their own stressors and life circumstances. Rarely does it benefit a team to *add* stress. Often, there are ways to express yourself calmly that address the issue without inflaming the situation. If the issue is serious, search online, use AI, or contact your human resources department for tips on how to have a productive conversation.

Early in my managing career, one of my staff members, without checking with me, sent an unnecessary email to leaders in Washington, D.C. that raised questions about how I was managing my project. This person thought sending the email evidenced independent thinking and initiative. Instead, it threatened to derail a million-plus-dollar project. My initial thought was to call the person on the carpet. "How could you do this? What were you thinking?" But I took some deep breaths and slowly realized that what looked like their error could be laid at *my* doorstep. What problems in our communication patterns led to this happening? Why was I not aware of their plans? Why did they not feel comfortable coming to me to check before sending the email? In the end, I said something like the following. "This was my fault, and I apologize. I should have been more aware of the pressures you were under and the plans for the email. It's also clear to me now that I failed to create an environment where you could send me a quick message to check in before you did something. So here are some ideas for how I plan to improve my accessibility and awareness of project issues. What do you think? I'm open to suggestions. I want to do better and support you better."

A principal investigator holds the ultimate responsibility for all parts of a grant submission or a funded project, including how the team behaves. This is true from a regulatory and compliance perspective. Embracing it as part of a management style follows suit. What I said during the above example was not perfect. But I surprised my staff member by presenting the mistake as my own. And that opened the door to an honest, problem-solving discussion about much more than one email.

The better you understand yourself, the easier it will be to remove your own emotions from conversations with your subordinates. You can only *learn* from the past, not transform it. So every constructive conversation should focus on potential *future change* in your subordinate's—or, better yet, your team's (including you)—behavior and how best to achieve that. Strong emotions can distort the bigger picture, potentially to the detriment of a conversation and relationship with an individual.

Chip and Dan Heath, in their book on behavior change, *The Power of Moments: Why Certain Experiences Have Extraordinary Impact* (2017, p. 123), outline four principles of supportive mentorship that boil down to the following mantra: "I have high expectations for you and I know you can meet them. So try this new challenge and if you fail, I'll help you recover." Endeavor to communicate this message implicitly and explicitly to those you manage. Your grant submissions and funded projects will benefit.

15.4.5 Embrace Diversity

The world is an uneven playing field. Institutions and structures across countries and all facets of life make achieving success more difficult for various groups and individuals. Yet when you recruit and retain people from groups that are underrepresented and, *at the same time*, value and draw out their identity-related knowledge, your team will be more effective. (One of the strengths of collaborative problem-solving during huddles is that it deliberately includes *all* ideas.) When you do this, your employees learn to embrace new perspectives and think in new ways. They also learn that this type of creativity and openness is sought after. An article in the *Harvard Business Review* (Ely & Thomas, 2020) provides more information about the benefits of diversity and includes research supporting why and how to incorporate it.

15.4.6 Help People Do What They Enjoy

One of the most successful strategies my teams and I have employed is to support group members in determining their strengths and what brings them joy in work. We then, to the extent possible, align their roles during proposal preparation and in a project with what they like and are good at. This exploration cannot occur overnight. Some individuals think they like or are good at one thing and over time learn (or the team learns) that something else is true. Maneuvering roles and positions requires flexibility that may not always be immediately available. But it is often possible to give people some tasks that align with their passions, even if those do not represent the bulk of what they do. This is one role of a manager: having ongoing discussions with employees about what satisfies them currently and their aspirations. You might be surprised how much an acknowledgment of someone's genuine desires can uplift a person and propel forward the work of proposal preparation and projects.

Like driving a car, effective people management is a valuable skill. Learning to do it well is difficult *and* rewarding. Just like with proposal writing, it offers a lifetime of opportunities for improvement. Embracing a growth mindset engages you in meaningful work that benefits you and everyone on your team. And, like driving, it takes you and your projects to new and exciting places. So get into the manager's seat, buckle up, and start the engine.

References

Ely, R.J. and Thomas, D.A. (2020, November-December). Getting Serious About Diversity: Enough Already with the Business Case. Harvard Business Review. https://hbr.org/2020/11/getting-serious-about-diversity-enough-already-with-the-business-case

Heath, C., & Heath, D. (2017). *The Power of Moments: Why Certain Experiences Have Extraordinary Impact*. Simon and Schster.

Chapter 16
Never Too Expert to Learn

I like the Japanese saying, “Even monkeys fall out of trees,” meaning that even experts make mistakes. I hope every proposal I participate in teaches me something. Here is a story from my fiftieth submission, coincidentally about falling, that makes me think I will never stop learning.

At that point in my career, I had significant skills under my belt. I understood and embraced the cognitive ease strategy. Grants I worked on were regularly funded. Yet the reviewer comments on this fiftieth application surprised me. As our team worked through how to respond to the critiques, the feedback taught me new ways to anticipate how reviewers think and perform their work. (See Chap. 13, Sect. 13.7.2 for more details on this particular application’s revision.)

The grant was about how to reduce the risk of falling for people living in nursing homes. We said we would judge the success of the study based on a rate of how often people fell, specifically the rate at which they had any fall at all. To do this, we would use a national dataset that contained different variables related to fall rates.

The first variable we mentioned in the proposal, in the one-page overview, was “falls with major injury.” This was *not* our outcome of interest. We brought it up because it highlights the potential drastic effects of falls. Falls with major injury are rare but severe. They result in trauma, such as a fractured arm or a broken hip. In our dataset, someone living in a nursing home is coded as “1” if they had a fall with major injury in the past three months and “0” if they did not have such a fall.

But the rarity of falls with major injury makes it difficult to use for a clinical trial such as the one we proposed. We thus chose a different variable to evaluate success: “any fall during an episode of care.” Fall severity does not matter for this. Even sliding gently but involuntarily out of bed and to the floor counts. Somone is coded “1” if they had *any* fall of *any* kind in the past three months and “0” if they never fell. As you can imagine, being coded 1 for this variable is much more common than for falls with major injury. In the population of interest, the fall rate for this variable was almost 20 times higher than for falls with major injury.

C. W. Hartmann, *Grant Writing Fundamentals Made Easy*,
https://doi.org/10.1007/978-3-032-35723-6_16

On the overview page, immediately after the mention of falls with major injury, we introduced any fall during an episode of care and had one sentence to describe the rates for any fall during an episode of care. And from then on, on that page, we discussed only any fall during an episode of care, because the success or failure of our intervention hinged on whether this improved.

But then in the background-providing section of the main narrative, we mentioned rates of falls with major injury numerous times to provide context, because an intervention that can improve this rare event is an effective intervention. And in our prior work, our intervention was successful at improving the rater of this rare event. The methods section then exclusively focused on any fall during an episode of care. As it turned out, all this back-and-forth confused reviewers considerably.

Because the proposal mentioned falls with major injury first on the overview page, reviewers remembered falls as being associated with major injury. They knew the grant was about falls, and the first type of fall we introduced was the kind with major injury, the rarer kind. After that, whenever they saw the word "fall," they thought "major injury" and "rare," even when the application used other words and explained another variable. They completely missed the introduction and repeated discussion of any fall during an episode of care. A tangential idea introduced as a comparison had already become, in reviewers' minds, the primary outcome.

Wow, was that a problem.

The main narrative pointed out how common any fall during an episode of care was. It described rates of its occurrence. A table with all outcome variables listed any fall during an episode of care in the top position. But in the reviewer comments, every reviewer complained about how *rare* the primary outcome was and how the proposal did not contain any data on rates of falls with major injury, even though this was how (they thought) we would measure success.

No, we did not include data on that, because falls with major injury was *not* the primary outcome variable. But every reviewer skipped over this fact.

The summary of the review group's discussion clearly indicated that no one interrupted the conversation to say, "Hold on. Falls with major injury *isn't* the primary outcome. Look at the middle of the overview page or on page two of the main narrative. They state the primary outcome is rates of any fall during an episode of care." Nope. Reviewers got on the major injury horse and rode it hard until the end.

It was a long ride. The misunderstanding about the primary outcome variable cascaded through many other parts of the proposal. They did not understand the rates. That called into question the study's feasibility. They thought the power calculation was wrong. They even questioned the literature review.

I believe reviewers missed the primary outcome variable partly because no heading in the main narrative included the name of the primary outcome or introduced text devoted exclusively to it. Overall, the narrative had too few headings, particularly in the section about background information. That section followed the 1–3-2 principle (see Chap. 7, Sect. 7.1), with important points at the beginning and end of paragraphs. But having those statements was not identical to having an entire paragraph focused on a single point, such as the primary outcome. In retrospect, we lumped too much information together, burying the most important information.

The longer a section of text is, the more cognitive strain it causes. In the revised application, each idea in the main narrative had its own heading. The primary outcome variable, of course, had one. But so did other ideas that could get lost. The background-providing text went from containing five headings to eight. If the text under a heading addressed more than one point or was more than two paragraphs long, we broke it up.

The original narrative also should have included a descriptive table for the rates of the primary outcome variable. Mentioning the rates in the text was not enough. Nobody noticed that. We needed a graphic to call attention to the data. In the revision, the rates were in a table next to the relevant section, with a descriptive title.

Naturally, we also removed all references to falls with major injury from the overview page.

The upside of the first submission's debacle was that responding to the reviewer comments required no new analyses. Everything the reviewers wanted to know was in the original submission. They simply had not noticed.

16.1 Final Thoughts

I think of writing grant proposals as similar to playing competitive sports. Both activities benefit from a commitment to advancing your skills. In both cases, you win some and lose some. And in both, the better you get, the more you are likely to win.

Improvement requires self-awareness and a willingness to seek out new ideas, try them, and study what happens. In my research projects, we consider everything a trial run. We never assume we have *the one right way* to do something. We give a concept, method, or process a shot, observe how it goes, and tweak or replace it as necessary. Even when all indicators point in positive directions, we revisit the issue from time to time. Different people bring suggestions, environments change, and we pick up lessons in other areas that we want to apply. Nothing is constant except change. So we adapt to improve.

For that reason, the grant writing journey humbles and amazes me. It embraces so many individuals and organizations with fantastic goals, so many alternative ways to solve a problem, so many efforts to cross the funding finish line. And there is never one correct answer, no perfect proposal, just the best attempt of that moment.

Yet throughout all the hard work, conversations, and collaborations, behind the adrenaline, frustration, and elation of the process, one question stands out for me as the driving engine for success. For whom do I write?

Asking myself that question changed my life. I hope it changes yours.

Index

C. W. Hartmann, *Grant Writing Fundamentals Made Easy*,
https://doi.org/10.1007/978-3-032-35723-6

FSC
www.fsc.org
MIX
Papier | Fördert gute Waldnutzung
FSC® C083411

Kolibri 360 GmbH
Ferdinand-Jühlke-Straße 7
99095 Erfurt, Deutschland
produktsicherheit@kolibri360.de